CAN'T SLEEP? ISSUES OF BEING AN INSOMNIAC

Edited by **Saddichha Sahoo**

Can't Sleep? Issues of Being an Insomniac
Edited by Saddichha Sahoo

Published by InTech

Janeza Trdine 9, 51000 Rijeka, Croatia

Publishing Process Manager Ivona Lovric

Technical Editor Teodora Smiljanic

Cover Designer InTech Design Team

Additional hard copies can be obtained from orders@intechopen.com

Can't Sleep? Issues of Being an Insomniac, Edited by Saddichha Sahoo
p. cm.
ISBN 978-953-51-0261-8

For EU product safety concerns:
IN TECH d.o.o., Prolaz Marije Krucifikse Kozulić 3, 51000 Rijeka, Croatia,
info@intechopen.com or visit our website at intechopen.com.

Meet the editor

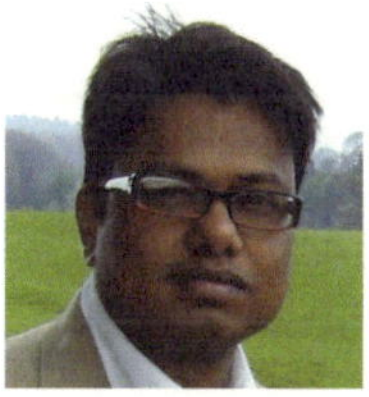

Dr Saddichha Sahoo, DPM MD, graduated in psychiatry from two premier institutions - Central Institute of Psychiatry and National Institute of Mental Health & Neurosciences, India. He is currently Clinical faculty at Department of Psychiatry, University of British Columbia, Vancouver. Dr Saddichha Sahoo main expertise and interest is in addiction psychiatry and psychopharmacology. He has published more than 75 scientific papers and edited 2 monographs and textbooks. He is on the editorial and review boards of several medical journals.

Contents

Preface

The word "insomnia" originates from the Latin "in" (no) and "somnus" (sleep). It is a disorder characterized by inability to fall asleep or a total lack of sleep. Being the first psychosomatic disorder to be described by Johann Heinroth in 1818, insomnia clinically presents as a subjective perception of dissatisfaction with the amount and/or quality of the sleep. The presenting complaints are often that of difficulties falling asleep in spite of being in bed, waking up several times during the night and having trouble going back to sleep, waking up too early in the morning or having an unrefreshing sleep.

Various studies have noted insomnia to be quite a common condition with symptoms present in about 33-50% of the adult population. The prevalence, however, ranges from 10 to 15% among the general population, with higher rates seen among divorced, separated, or widowed people, older ages, female gender, White population, and in the presence of a co-morbid medical or psychiatric illness. About 30% of all adults complain of occasional insomnia and 10% of chronic insomnia, of whom 40% may have an underlying psychiatric illness. Despite these high prevalence rates, evidence suggests that insomnia is mostly under recognized, under-diagnosed, and under-treated, with the condition continuing to remain persistent in most individuals over follow-up intervals of one to several years.

Chronic insomnia represents a more complex condition than acute insomnia, which may be transient. Patients with chronic insomnia usually have accompanying daytime impairment of cognition, mood, or performance that impacts not only the patient and his family, but also affects friends, coworkers, and caretakers. Insomnia patients are more likely to visit hospitals and physicians, have increased absenteeism, make errors or have accidents at work, and have more fatal road accidents. There is also an increased risk for depression, anxiety, substance use, suicide, and possible immune dysfunction. It is imperative that clinicians remain alert to these possible individual and societal risks during the evaluation.

This book deals with several issues that are pertinent to the clinician and researcher in insomnia practice. The first chapter deals with the current knowledge of the epidemiology and risk factors for developing insomnia. A review of medications that may also induce insomnia follows which details out the common mistakes that a clinician does while examining a patient with insomnia. Since insomnia is directly linked to issues such as productivity and quality of life, comprehensive reviews cover these subjects. The diagnosis and management of insomnia is detailed out next with a brief and lucid description of barbiturates which are often used in the treatment of insomnia.

Dr. Saddichha Sahoo, DPM MD,
Clinical Fellow, Dept of Psychiatry, University of British Columbia,
Vancouver, BC,
Canada

Part 1

Epidemiology and Risk Factors

1

Epidemiology of Insomnia: Prevalence and Risk Factors

Claudia de Souza Lopes[1],
Jaqueline Rodrigues Robaina[1] and Lúcia Rotenberg[2]
[1]*Institute of Social Medicine, State University of Rio de Janeiro (IMS-UERJ)*
[2]*Oswaldo Cruz Institute, Oswaldo Cruz Foundation (IOC-FIOCRUZ)*
Brazil

1. Introduction

Insomnia is among the most prevalent health complaints, with approximately 10 to 15% of the general population suffering regularly from it and about 25 to 35% presenting transient or occasional insomnia (Ancoli-Israel & Roth, 1999; Ohayon, 2002; Morin et al., 2006; Doghramji, 2006; LeBlanc et al., 2009). However, many questions remain unanswered with regard to our understanding of insomnia and prevalence estimates vary because of inconsistent definitions and diagnostic criteria. In addition, the use of baseline and follow-up assessments to establish incidence and remission rates can be problematic because of the wide spectrum of insomnia duration (e.g., a positive finding of insomnia at baseline and 1-year follow-up may reflect unremitting chronic insomnia or 2 episodes of transient insomnia) (Roth, 2001; Young, 2005).

The elderly in particular are affected by insomnia, and it has been shown that women are more likely to have sleep difficulties than men. Although insomnia can be a primary condition, and can coexist with other disorders or be considered secondary to these disorders, the mechanisms producing it are not clearly defined (Doghramji, 2006).

Insomnia can be brought on by psychosocial causes, co-morbid medical disorders, abuse of alcohol or other substances. The relationship between insomnia and psychosocial and medical conditions is believed to be reciprocal; each condition may cause, maintain, and even exacerbate the other.

2. Prevalence of insomnia

There is no consensus for classification used in defining insomnia in terms of its symptoms, frequency and severity. These variations of the definition and population studied determine the wide variation in the estimated prevalence (Ohayon, 2002; Mai & Buysse, 2008; Roth et al., 2011).

Various are the concepts used to define insomnia, which range from the concept of "unsatisfactory sleep" developed by the American Medicine Institute in 1979, to the International Classification of Sleep Disorders (ASDA, 1990) definition according to which insomnia corresponds to the complaint of insufficient sleep almost every night or by being tired after the usual sleep time. The three main diagnostic manuals, International Classification of Sleep Disorders (ICSD-2) (American Academy of Sleep Medicine, 2005), Diagnostic and Statistic Manual (DSM IVTR) (American Psychiatric Association, 2000), and International Classification of Disease (ICD-10) (World Health Organization, 1992), vary in their approach to defining insomnia.

Another important source of variation streams from the need of hiring professional interviewers or laborious instruments for its measure according to the most commonly used criteria. Besides, the frequent association of insomnia and mental disorders, results in a wide variation between the concepts used and the means to measure primary insomnia.

As a result of these differences in insomnia case definitions, estimates of insomnia prevalence have varied widely, from 10–40% (Bixler et al., 1979; Ford & Kamerow, 1989; Kuppermann et al., 1995; Üstun et al., 1996; Simon & Von Korff, 1997; Ancoli-Israel & Roth, 1999; Léger et al., 2000; Ohayon e Roth, 2001; Ohayon, 2002; Li et al., 2002; Rocha et al., 2002; Pires et al., 2007; Roth et al., 2011). Given all the information available, the prevalence of insomnia symptoms may be estimated at 30% and specific insomnia disorders at 5-10% (Roth et al., 2007; Mai & Buysse, 2008).

A third of the Americans have reported one or more insomnia symptoms: difficulty in falling asleep, difficulty to maintain sleep, waking up very early, and in some cases, a non-restorative or a bad quality sleep, in a study by the National Sleep Foundation in conjunction with the Gallup Organization, which objective was, from telephone interviews examine the prevalence and nature of the difficulty in sleeping (Ancoli-Israel & Roth, 1999). More recently, the America Insomnia Survey conducted among 10,094 health care plan subscribers, assessed insomnia using the Brief Insomnia Questionnaire (BIQ). The questionnaire, developed for the study generated diagnoses of insomnia according to the definitions and criteria of the SDM-IV_TR, ICD-10 and RDC/ICSD-2 systems (Summers et al., 2006). This study found that insomnia prevalence estimates varied widely, from 22.1% for DSM-IV-TR to 3.9% for ICD-10 criteria; the RDC/ICSD-2 estimate was 14.7% (Roth et al., 2011).

Ohayon e Roth (2001) in a transversal study with a representative sample of 24,600 individuals of the populations of France, United Kingdom, Germany, Italy, Portugal and Spain, 15 years old or more, found a 10.1% prevalence for difficulty in going to sleep and 22.2% to mantaining sleep, with a frequency of three or more times a week. When using the DSM-IV criteria to diagnose insomnia (complaint of difficulty in falling asleep or to maintain sleep or of a non-restorative sleep, for at least one month, causing clinically significant distress or impairment in the individual) this prevalence is 11.1%. Also in France, Léger et al. (2000), in a sample of 12,778 people, reported a prevalence of 21% and 16%, in falling asleep and maintaining sleep, respectively, and 19% of insomnia, according to the DSM-IV criteria.

In a study in the city of Hong Kong, where the definition used was the positive response (sometimes or always) at least three times a week in the last month, the prevalence found in 9,851 individuals between 18 and 65 years old was of 4.4% for difficulty in falling asleep, 6.9% maintaining sleep after being interrupted and 4% for early morning awakening. The prevalence of insomnia (considering a positive answer to any of these questions) was 11.9% (Li et al., 2002).

In Latin America, there are few studies on sleep disorders and its occurrence in the population. In Brazil, Rocha et al. (2002), in a population-study of 1,221 individuals in a city in Minas Gerais State (Bambuí), found 35.4% prevalence of insomnia in the adult population (more than 18 years old). The most common complaint was of intermediate insomnia (27.3%); followed by initial insomnia (18.3%) and final insomnia (14.3%), with a frequency of three or more times a week, during the last month. In São Paulo State, Pires and collaborators (2007) performed a study to compare prevalence of insomnia complaints and sleep habits among women of more than 20 years old in a general population sample, between the years 1987 and 1995. The criterion used was frequency, where those who answered questions about insomnia "of three to six times a week" or "daily" were considered insomniacs. The results were: for difficulty in falling asleep 17.2% (in 1987) and 23.5% (in 1995) and for difficulty in maintaining sleep 18.6% and 29.8% (in 1987 and 1995, respectively). Marchi and collaborators (2004) in a study conducted with 833 women between 18 and 90 years old and that used DSM-IV criteria to diagnose insomnia, observed prevalence of 35,4% among women of a city in São Paulo State (São José do Rio Preto).

In order to understand the high prevalence of insomnia and to provide evidence for a better treatment or management of that in the health care, epidemiological studies in this area have focused on the complex pathways of the determination of insomnia. A new generation of studies has investigated which factors have been implicated in its development and persistence.

3. Risk factors for insomnia

3.1 Socio-demographic and economic factors

Factors most commonly associated to insomnia are: gender, age, marital status, income, educational level, and race/ethnicity. Sleep disorders affect women and men differently and may have different manifestations and prevalences (Philips at al., 2008).

A consistent finding in literature is the higher prevalence of insomnia among women than in men (Breslau et al., 1996; Léger et al., 2000; Sutton et al., 2002; Ohayon, 2002; Ohayon & Partinen, 2002; Ohayon & Hong, 2002), there being few studies that observed higher prevalence in men (Kim et al., 2000).

A meta-analysis of more than 29 studies and 1,265,015 individuals showed that women have a 41% higher risk (95% CI 1.28–1.55) of developing insomnia than men (Zhang & Wing, 2006). In another study, data from the *National Sleep Foundation* showed that 57% of women suffer one or more insomnia symptoms at least some nights a week (National Sleep Foundation, 2005). Women reported a larger number of insomnia symptoms, with daytime consequences, dissatisfaction with sleep and having a diagnosis of insomnia when compared to males. The woman/man ratio for insomnia symptoms is about 4:1, increasing with age (Ohayon, 2002).

Léger et al. (2000) demonstrated that the more restrictive the criteria for insomnia, the more important the difference between sexes. The prevalence, when the criteria evaluate only one complaint of insomnia is 78% among women and 68% among men. When using DSM-IV criteria, prevalence is 22% among women and 14% among men, and if criteria include more than one complaint of sleep disorders with daily consequences (criteria for severe insomnia), prevalence is 12% in women and 6.3% in men.

Another study identified some risk factors specific to gender. Low educational level and retirement were associated to a higher risk of insomnia in men, while being divorced or widow, housewife and sleep in a noisy atmosphere, were associated to a higher risk of insomnia in women (Li et al., 2002).

The reasons why women are more affected than men are not well known. Evidences suggest that insomnia may occur in association to hormone changes that are unique to women, such as those accompanying them during menopause. Although the relationship between hormone levels and sleep is complex, it seems that there is a correlation between the decrease in circulating estrogens and progesterone and an increase of insomnia prevalence (Krystal, 2003). The decrease of complaints during hormone therapy may be an indicator that its occurrence is in part due to the fall of female sexual hormones that occur at menopause (Polo-Kantola et al., 1998; Sarti et al., 2005).

Another possible explanation for this difference between sexes is given by the fact that women present a higher prevalence of mental disorders, especially depression and anxiety (Li et al., 2002), which would increase the risk of insomnia. Another hypothesis is that women would be more sensitive to the methods of measuring insomnia, because culturally women are allowed greater freedom to show their emotions while men tend to hide or not to admit them (Panda-Moreno et al., 2001).

Most epidemiologic studies report a higher prevalence of insomnia symptoms with age (Bixler et al., 1979; Vela-Bueno et al., 1999; Léger et al., 2000; Kim et al., 2000), but some authors associate this increase in prevalence to factors that would contribute to a worse quality sleep and not to age *per se* (Lamberg, 2003). With age, psychological and medical problems and medicines used in these treatments would cause a decline in sleep quality (Lee et al., 2008).

Sutton et al. (2002) in a study conducted in a representative sample of the Canadian population over 15 years old did not find a significant association between age and insomnia. For these and other authors, insomnia should not be considered as a component of the aging process and studies should consider the multifactorial aetiology. In this age group, individuals present a higher difficulty to adjust to new changes in life, e.g. retirement, change of address, loss of family members (Panda-Moreno et al., 2001). Another explanation is a growth in circulatory, digestive and respiratory diseases (Ohayon e Zulley, 2001), changes in circadian rhythms (Roth & Roehrs, 2003), allergies, migraines, rheumatic disorders (Ohayon e Zulley, 2001), etc. All these factors show a significant association to insomnia.

In some studies (Pallesen et al., 2001; Ohayon e Partinen, 2002), the prevalence of insomnia did not behave as expected. Prevalence of initial insomnia was higher in the younger groups, a result that is probably related to group lifestyle (e.g. staying up until late on weekends) or to circadian factors. Ohayon e Zulley (2001) report that among the youth, stress would have a more important role in prevalence of insomnia than in the elderly, when probably physical illnesses would be more significant.

Studies that examined the association between marital status and insomnia generally report a higher prevalence in separated/divorced individuals or widowed (Ohayon et al., 1997; Léger et al., 2000; Li et al., 2002) when compared to single or married.

In Brazil, results of investigations conducted by Rocha et al. (2002) confirm this association. Widowed (OR = 2.3; 95% CI 1.5–3.5) and separated/divorced (OR = 2.2; 95% CI 1.2–4.2) were more likely to suffer from insomnia when compared to married individuals.

Prevalence of insomnia is higher in individuals with low income and in those with low literacy (Bixler et al., 1979; Li et al., 2002). However, further studies using multivariate analysis did not identify low-income and low literacy as independent risk factors for insomnia (Ohayon et al., 1997). One hypothesis to explain these results is that, among individuals with low literacy and low income, these factors could reflect additional social disadvantage such as unemployment and poor living conditions in general (Pallesen et al., 2001), which could feed daily stress or lead to insomnia (Kim et al., 2000).

The high occurrence of physical and mental health problems could be a possible explanation, presented by Rocha and collaborators (2002), to a higher prevalence of insomnia among individuals with low socio-economic development.

Another SDE factor studied is race. Prevalence of insomnia is generally higher among blacks as compared to whites (Bixler et al., 2002). Folley et al. (1999), in a cohort study among elderly (65 years old or more), with a three year follow-up, found that the incidence of insomnia was higher in black women (19%), followed by white men and women with 14% and black males (12%). Among blacks, women had a higher risk of developing insomnia (OR = 1.58; 95% CI 1.03–2.41), when compared to men. Among whites, risk of developing insomnia did not differ between male and female (OR = 0.77; 95% CI 0.50–1.20).

In a Brazilian study conducted at Bambuí (Rocha et al., 2002) prevalence was higher in white individuals (52.8%), followed by mulattos/browns (44.3%) and blacks (2.9%), but the univariate analysis performed found no statistically significant association between insomnia and race, when comparing white with mulattos/browns (OR = 1.0; 95% CI 0.80–1.3) and blacks (OR = 1.4; 95% CI 0.6–3.0).

3.2 Physical and mental morbidity

Links between poor physical health and insomnia have repeatedly been demonstrated, (Moffitt et al., 1991; Sutton et al., 2001; Martikainen et al., 2003; Roth & Roehrs, 2003; Buysse, 2004; Ohayon & Bader, 2010) as many diseases involve pain and/or distress that can interfere with sleep. Using data from the 2002 Canadian Community Health Survey (CCHS): Mental Health and Well-being, Tjpkema (2005), reported that over 20% of people with asthma, arthritis/rheumatism, back problems or diabetes reported insomnia, compared with around 12% of people who did not have these conditions. After adjustment for demographic, socio-economic, lifestyle and several psychological factors, the conditions that remained independently related to insomnia were fibromyalgia, arthritis/rheumatism, back problems, migraine, heart disease, cancer, chronic bronchitis/emphysema/chronic obstructive pulmonary disease, stomach/intestinal ulcers, and bowel disorders. On the other hand, associations between insomnia and asthma, high blood pressure, diabetes and the effects of stroke disappeared.

Despite the importance of physical morbidity on the aetiology and maintenance of insomnia, emotional and mental disorders appear to play an even more important role on that (Breslau et al., 1996; Li et al., 2002). In fact, studies have reported that insomnia secondary to a psychiatric disorder is the most common diagnostic entity in 30%–50% of patients (Coleman et al., 1982).

As with physical morbidity, the relationship between insomnia and mental disorders is known to be bidirectional. Insomnia can be both a risk factor (Lustberg & Reynolds, 2000) and a consequence of depression (Lustberg & Reynolds, 2000; Roberts et al., 2000), of anxiety disorders and abuse of alcohol and other substances (LeBlanc et al., 2009).

The association between insomnia and major depressive episodes has been constantly reported: individuals with insomnia are more likely to have a major depressive illness. Longitudinal studies have shown that the persistence of insomnia is associated with the appearance of a new depressive episode.

The presence of insomnia symptoms was reported in 80% of individuals with a major depressive diagnosis, and levels close to 90% among patients with diagnosis of anxiety disorder (Ohayon, 2002). Research by Breslau et al. (1996) among young adults (21 to 30 years old) in Michigan, USA, found, after adjusting to gender, that individuals with history of insomnia in the last weeks presented four times higher chances to be diagnosed with depression (OR = 3.9; 95% CI 2.22–7.0) and twice higher for any kind of anxiety (OR = 1.97; 95% CI 1.08–3.6).

LeBlanc et al. (2009) in a population-based longitudinal study among adults participants from a larger epidemiologic study conducted in Quebec, Canada, found that, when compared to good sleepers, insomnia syndrome incident cases presented higher depressive and anxiety symptoms at baseline.

Individuals with sleep problems have significantly higher levels of common mental disorders. Research conducted by Üstün et al. (1996), in 15 cities in 14 different countries with outpatients between 15 and 65 years old, showed that, after deleting the item relating to sleep in the questionnaire ("the last two weeks, you have lost much sleep over worry?"), the General Health Questionnaire (GHQ-12) score - screening tool for these disorders - was twice greater for these patients with sleep problems when compared to those without sleep problems. In the same study, patients who reported positively for at least one question about insomnia complaints, the relative risk for depression was 9.0 (95% CI 7.7-10.5) and 3.9 for generalized anxiety (95% CI 3.3-4.6).

Research using data from the 2002 Canadian Community Health Survey (CCHS): Mental Health and Well-being showed mental and emotional health to be strongly associated with insomnia (Johnson & Breslau, 2001; Sutton et al., 2001; Ohayon, 2002; Martikainen et al., 2003; Ohayon & Roth, 2003). Around a third of people who reported having had an anxiety or mood disorder in the past year had insomnia, compared to 12% of those who did not have such disorders.

More recently, a population-based study conducted among 5,001 Chinese adults in Hong-Kong, showed that higher scores of depression and anxiety (Hospital Anxiety and Depression Scale - HADS) and poor mental health component of quality of life measures (QoL) were significantly associated with insomnia (Wong & Fielding, 2011).

3.3 Alcohol and other substances

Several studies have reported sleep problems associated with the use of several illicit drugs, and the vast majority of alcoholic patients entering treatment reported insomnia-related symptoms, such as difficulty falling and maintaining sleep (Mahfoud et al., 2009; Tjepkma,

2005). For example, the prevalence of insomnia ranged from 36 to 72 percent in patients admitted for alcoholism treatment, depending on sample characteristics and instruments used to measure insomnia (Foster et al., 2000; Brower et al., 2001).

Alcohol, which is a sedating agent, can aid the onset of sleep. However, it can also lead to increased arousal later in the sleep cycle, and with continued use, its benefits as a sleep aid is reduced (Quereshi & Lee-Chiong, 2004).

According to the results of the CCHS, 16% of frequent heavy drinkers reported insomnia, compared to 13% of those who were not frequent heavy drinkers, and this association persisted even after adjustment for other factors. In the same study, they found that about one in five (18%) people who used cannabis, but no other illicit drugs, reported insomnia at least once a week, significantly higher than the 13% reported by those who did not use illicit drugs or used them less frequently (Tjepkema, 2005).

In a Chinese population-based study, those consuming alcohol four to seven times a week had higher adjusted odds (OR = 4.7; 95% CI 1.6-13.4) of reporting insomnia than those who never consumed alcohol (Wong & Fielding, 2011).

Besides alcohol consumption, caffeine, drug withdrawal, and use of stimulants are also associated to sleep disruption (Ramakrishnan & Scheid, 2007).

Smoking was also positively related to difficulties in falling asleep and estimated sleep latency (Janson et al., 1995). Similar results were described by Philips and Danner (1995), who observed that cigarette smokers were significantly more likely than non-smokers to report difficulties in falling asleep, maintaining sleep as well as daytime sleepiness.

3.4 Chronic pain

Disrupted sleep pattern or insomnia is one of the most prevalent complaints among persons with chronic pain conditions and is associated with pain discomfort. As the other factors evaluated, the relationship between chronic pain and insomnia is believed to be reciprocal (McCracken & Iverson, 2002; Wilson et al., 2002; Benca et al., 2004; Lautenbacher et al., 2006; Gupta et al., 2007; Gureje, 2007; Roth et al., 2007; Goral et al., 2010).

Using data from the Israel National Health Survey (INHS) conducted in 2003–2004 on a representative sample (N = 4,859) of the adult Israeli population, Goral et al., (2010) found that chronic pain was associated with both sleep problems and increased health care utilization even for individuals with no psychiatric comorbidity. Sleep difficulties but not health care utilization rates were more pronounced in the comorbid group compared to the chronic pain only group.

3.5 Menopause

Insomnia is the most frequent sleep disorder in postmenopause. Studies demonstrated that women in perimenopause and postmenopause present a higher sleep latency, difficulty in maintaining and are less satisfied with sleep when compared to those in premenopause (Landis & Moe, 2004).

Hormone changes, depressive states related to this period of life or to vasomotor symptoms (hot flashes and/or nocturia), besides chronic pain are some of the probable causes of insomnia associated to menopause. Some studies refer to difficulty in determining if changes in sleep are due to aging or to menopausal status (Shaver & Zenk, 2000; Campos et al., 2005; Pérez et al., 2009).

Insomnia during menopause is frequently attributed to the heat waves. According to the majority of studies, it is more strongly associated with vasomotor symptoms, probably due to the cascade of symptoms: hot flashes and sweating at night generating insomnia, and, consequently, irritability and fatigue the following day (Pedro et al., 2003; Landis & Moe, 2004).

Prevalence of insomnia as a menopause symptom is relatively high, as shown in studies:

An Australian population-based follow-up study (Melbourne Women's Midlife Health Project) with 438 women (from 45 to 55 years old) followed for seven years analyzed changes in symptoms of menopause in terms of prevalence and severity. An increased prevalence of insomnia in time after menopause was observed. Thus, the reporting of sleep difficulties was observed in 38%, 43% and 45% of women with one, two and three years of post-menopause, respectively (Dennerstein et al., 2000).

In Spain, a sectional study, accomplished in 2006, with 10,514 women between 45 to 65 years old, observed a prevalence of insomnia of 45.7%. Prevalence of insomnia was of 37.5% among women in perimenopause and 49.4% in postmenopause (Pérez et al., 2009).

Another study that addresses insomnia in relation to the menopause transition was conducted in the Netherlands, with 2,450 women between 47 and 54 years old. Prevalence of insomnia in premenopause, perimenopause and postmenopause was of 37%, 47% and 60%, respectively. The crude odds ratios were: 0.99 (women in perimenopause compared to those in premenopause), 1.34 (women in postmenopause compared to those in perimenopause), and 2.06 (women in postmenopause compared to those in premenopause) (Maartens et al., 2001).

In a cohort study in Korea with 2,497 women between 40 and 60 years old, the prevalence of insomnia increases significantly in the transition from premenopause (7.3%) to perimenopause (15.9%) and to postmenopause (19.7%). The association between insomnia and the transition to menopause remained even after adjusting for age, education, income, marital status, physical illness, depression, and BMI, with ORs from 2.1 to 1.4 for perimenopause and postmenopause when compared to premenopausal women (Shin et al., 2005).

In Brazil, a household survey in Campinas (São Paulo State) in 1997, with 456 women, between 45-60 years old assessed the existence and frequency of symptoms - hot flashes, sweating, palpitations and dizziness (vasomotor symptoms) - in 4 weeks preceding the survey (replies: never, less than three times a day, from three to ten times a day and 11 times or more). The instrument also included psychological symptoms such as nervousness, irritability, headaches, depression and insomnia. Insomnia was one of the most prevailing among psychological symptoms. The percentage of insomniac women was 54.5%, prevalence which grew as the state of menopause, being 40.6% in premenopause, 55.9% in perimenopause and 61.1% in postmenopause (Pedro et al., 2003).

Still in Brazil, the evaluation of postmenopausal sleep quality (defined as "sleep badly" always or most times), with 271 women between 35 and 65 years old, treated at private clinics or at school-hospitals in São Paulo city showed prevalence of 18.6% in premenopause, 37.5% in perimenopause, 28.9% in natural postmenopause and 38.9% in post-surgical menopause (Souza et al., 2005). In this study peri and surgical postmenopause were associated to "sleeping badly" (OR = 2.63; 95% CI 1.25-5.51 and OR = 2.78; 95% CI 1.18-6.60), respectively. Natural postmenopause and the use of HRT were not statistically significantly associated to "sleeping badly".

Study results show an improvement in subjective sleep quality (Montplaisir et al., 2001; Saletu-Zyhlarz et al., 2003), improved psychological well-being (Purdie et al., 1995) and the diminishment of hot spells (Purdie et al., 1995; Montplaisir et al., 2001) with the use of hormone replacement. In contrast, a recent study accomplished by Kalleinen (2008) shows that although the hormone replacement restores hormone levels after menopause, it offers no advantages as regards sleep deprivation.

The lack of consistency among the results of the studies has been attributed mainly to differences in protocols used in studies based on use of hormone therapy, duration of treatment, age and symptoms of the subjects and type of menopause (natural or surgical) (Kalleinen, 2008).

3.6 Psychosocial factors

One of the most consistent findings in the literature is the association between psychosocial factors and incidence and persistence of insomnia. The huge changes in the demography and economy that occurred mainly in the last decades worldwide have a parallel in the people's lifestyle, the way people interact in their work, family disruption, lack of social support, among others. These changes have been implicated to the high levels of stress and sleep problems found in the studies in this area.

3.6.1 Stress and stressful life events

Stress is an important factor related to insomnia. Stressful situations increase the psychological and physiological activation in response to increased environmental demands. Such activation is incompatible with deactivation which is the main feature of sleep. Thus, the scientific literature confirms the common sense notion that stress *disrupts* sleep (Akersted, 2006). On the other hand, the relationship between stress and sleep has to be evaluated in the light of its bidirectionality. In fact, stress impairs sleep quality, and chronic sleep difficulty is likely to become a stressor in itself, thus promoting a vicious circle of stress and insomnia (Akerstedt, 2006).

The occurrence stressful life events (SLE) has been shown to be strongly associated to chronic insomnia (Healey et al., 1981; Kim et al., 2000; Ohayon & Zulley, 2001; Robaina et al., 2009) and is mediated by certain personality factors. Insomniacs tend to be unhappier in interpersonal relationships and have a relatively low self-esteem, having inadequate *coping* mechanisms to deal with stress (Ohayon & Hong, 2002; Basta et al., 2007). However, in the majority of cases, primary insomnia (aetiology that is not related to another mental disorder, medical condition or substance dependence) may be induced by a stress situation, such as: withdrawal of a family member, sadness, loss or stress at work, economic difficulty, surgical intervention, etc, that would occupy the individual's mind while trying to sleep (LeBlanc et al., 2009; Kim et al., 2011). According to Yaniv (2004), about 74% of individuals that have sleep difficulties remember stressing life experiences associated to the beginning of their insomnia (e.g. personal losses, illnesses, marriage conflicts, etc). Once surpassed the critical period of occurrence of the triggering event, the subsequent insomnia could be another stress factor, since it affects activities related to everyday life (e.g. increasing the risk of losing one's job due to the impairment of efficiency in the work environment). Over time the effect of stress could be amplified resulting in a vicious circle, which would increase the levels of insomnia and stress.

Based on data from the 2002 Canadian Community Health Survey (CCHS), Tjepkema (2005) found that close to a quarter (23%) of people who described most of their days as being either "quite a bit" or "extremely" stressful reported insomnia and this was more than twice the percentage for people who reported little or no stress. According to the author, this difference persists even when physical and emotional/mental health along with socio-demographic, economic and lifestyle factors, were taken into account. Another finding reported is that the type of stress also made a difference; people whose main source of stress was a physical health problem, the death of a close relative, an emotional/mental health problem, personal/family responsibilities or problems in personal relationship had higher rates of insomnia compared with the overall rate.

Among Americans who suffered with occasional insomnia, the following events were described as the cause of difficulty to sleep: work stress (28% of individuals), family stress (20%) and death in the family (12%), according to research accomplished by the *National Sleep Foundation* together with the *Gallup Organization* (Ancoli-Israel & Roth, 1999).

A research conducted in Germany among the general population aged 15 years old or more, showed that individuals who reported having experienced some stressful event in the past year had more chance of being dissatisfied with their sleep, even after adjusting to age and sex (OR = 1.8; 95% CI 1.4-2.5). The chance of referring to dissatisfaction with sleep was greater among the people who perceived themselves suffering a high degree of stress (OR = 2.2; 95% CI 1.5-3.2), followed by those who presented a medium level of stress (OR = 1.5; 95% CI 1.0-2.1), when compared to individuals that did not report stress (Ohayon & Zulley, 2001).

In Brazil, a study conducted by Robaina and cols (2009) showed an important association between SLE and insomnia complaints of auxiliary nurses at a university hospital. The SLE associated to complaints of frequent insomnia were: "disrupter of relationship" (OR = 3.32; 95% CI 1.90-5.78), "serious health problems" (OR = 2.82; 95% CI 1.73-4.58); "serious financial difficulties" (OR = 2.38; 95% CI 1.46-3.88), and "forced change of residence" (OR = 1.97; 95% CI 1.02-3.79).

3.6.2 Job stress and other work characteristics

Occupational risk factors, such as shift work, job strain and number of work hours can also be linked to insomnia (Härmä et al., 1998; Nakata et al., 2001).

An essential aspect to be considered in this context is the stress originated by the work environment. There is widespread evidence that job stress can act as a risk factor for insomnia, as shown by several epidemiological studies on psychosocial job characteristics (Schnall et al., 2000; Akersted, 2006).

An important theoretical model for evaluating psychosocial conditions at the workplace is the demand-control model, designed by Karasek (1979). It considers the interrelationship between two components in the work process: (i) psychological demands: work overload, difficulties and little time available for the completion of work amongst others, and (ii) control: autonomy over one's own tasks, the possibility of using, developing, and acquiring new abilities (Karasek & Theorell, 1990). The perception of social support (from supervisor and from colleagues) was later included in this model by Johnson and Hall (1988). This dimension refers to the emotional integration, trust and assistance in performing, and was supposed to act as a moderator in the relationship between stress at work and health. The complete model is commonly referred to as the Demand-Control-Support model (Hausser et al., 2010).

A strong link between stressful working conditions - as measured by the demand-control model - and sleep was described by Kalimo and cols (2000) in a sample of 3,079 middle-aged working men in Finland. According to this study, the combination of high demands and low control (usually called *job strain*) was associated to a 30% prevalence of sleep disturbances, whereas a 5% prevalence of sleep disturbances was observed in the low demand-high control group. The study by Ota et al. (2005) also showed high job strain to be related to insomnia in 1,081 middle-aged workers in Japan.

The risk of insomnia increased with a higher degree of job strain, and decreased with a higher degree of job control in a sample of office workers. The combination of high strain with low degree of control or social support had an approximately three times higher risk of insomnia, as compared to that of low job strain with high degree of control or support (Nomura et al., 2009).

The analysis of the demand and control scores separately showed that only the demand was significantly related to disturbed sleep in a sample of healthy employed men and women in Sweden (Akerstedt et al., 2002a). Interestingly, the inclusion of an item corresponding to the inability to stop thinking about work during free time yield the highest OR, and forced work demands out of the regression.

In addition, an important connection between social support and sleep was also observed by Akerstedt et al. (2002b), as the lack of social support at the workplace was a risk indicator for disturbed sleep, not feeling rested and difficulties awakening.

Another theory-based conceptual job stress model for evaluating the relationship between job stress and sleep disturbances is the so-called effort-reward imbalance (ERI) model (Siegrist, 1996). According to this model, the imbalance perceived between these two dimensions (excess effort put in to fulfil work tasks and gaining insufficient recognition for this) generates stressful situations (Siegrist, 1996; Peter & Siegrist, 2000). The reward component corresponds to the returns that a worker expects to gain financially (adequate salary), self-esteem (respect and support), and occupational status (perspectives of promotion, work stability and social status). Effort takes into account the demands and obligations perceived by the worker (Peter & Siegrist, 2000). A third dimension was incorporated in the ERI model, called "over-commitment with work". This is defined as a set of attitudes, behaviour, and emotions that reflect excessive effort in conjunction with a strong need for recognition and esteem (Peter & Siegrist, 2000). The imbalance between exerted effort and expected reward, mediated by over-commitment with work, would potentially be the highest risk factor for falling ill.

There is increasing evidence for the relevance of the ERI in relation to sleep disturbances. Peter and collaborators (1998) found that ERI was associated with sleep disturbances in a group of female transport workers. According to Fahlén et al. (2006), higher levels of exposure for the ERI components are associated with increased prevalence of sleep disturbances in a subset of the WOLF (WOrk, Lipids, Fibrinogen) cohort study. For women, the strongest association was seen between high effort/reward ratio and sleep disturbances (PR = 4.13, 95% CI 1.62-10.5), and between high effort and sleep disturbances (PR = 4.04, 95% CI 1.53-10.7). For men, the high over-commitment and fatigue (not sleep disturbances) yielded the most obvious association.

Actually, the relevance of over-commitment was described by Kudielka et al. (2004) in a longitudinal cohort study on employers from two German companies. The authors observed that workers were 1.7 times more likely to report disturbed sleep per standard deviation increase in over-commitment. Gender-stratified analyses revealed that higher over-commitment was associated with unfavourable sleep in men, while in women poor sleep was related to lower reward.

To Akerstedt (2006), it is possible that work demands in themselves are not the most important elements in terms of insomnia, but the concern or the anticipation of the work demands, which, in this author's view was corroborated by the results of studies with techniques of polysomnography.

In a series of cross-sectional and prospective studies on a representative sample of Danish employers, Rugulies and collaborators (2009) observed that ERI was a risk factor for the development of sleep disturbances among men, whereas among women, the association between ERI and sleep was restricted to the cross-sectional sample.

In this context, a new approach was described by Ota et al. (2005). The authors showed that the simultaneous use of two stress models (demand-control and effort-reward imbalance) is more useful in the identification of workers at risk of insomnia than the use of each model separately. In a recent prospective study, Ota et al. (2009) observed that reward from work effort and sufficient support at work assist recovery from insomnia (at baseline), while over-commitment and high job strain cause future onset of insomnia.

Another prospective longitudinal study (five-year follow-up) on work and sleep showed that "having to hurry" was the main psychosocial occupational factor associated to sleep disturbances in a random sample of employed men and women. In this study, the authors also identified other risk factors for the changes in sleep, after controlling gender and age, namely shift work, long weekly hours and vibration in the work environment (Ribet & Derriennic, 1999).

Other relevant aspects of work environment have been associated to sleep disturbances. In a study with a representative sample of the Swedish population, Akerstedt (2002) observed the following work features as significant predictors of disturbed sleep: hectic work, physically strenuous work, and shift work. Amongst these aspects, shift work is the most investigated given its striking effects the quality of sleep (Akerstedt, 2003).

In fact, shift work is a well-known occupational risk factor for insomnia. The term *shift work* refers to hours of employment outside the typical day schedule from 8 a.m. to 5 p.m. on Monday to Friday, thus referring to work during non-standard hours, including night work and/or work on weekends (Presser, 2003).

There is emerging evidence from studies on insomnia that individuals with shift work are at a higher risk for lack of sleep (Ohayon, 2002). Such evidence is added to those observed in the field of occupational health. In fact, of all of the occupational factors, shift work is the most investigated given its striking consequences to quality of sleep (Akerstedt, 2003).

The consequences of work hours are clearly related to the design of the shift system. Comparisons of work schedules performed by Härmä et al. (1998) showed that insomnia complaints were more common in rotating shift work, and in irregular shift work than in day work. Also, the effects of physical activity and alcohol consumption differed for different shift schedules. Considering the diversity of shift schemes, the most important in terms of effects over sleep is the nightshift. Night work has repeatedly been associated with sleep problems, when compared to other types of shift (Ingre & Akersted, 2004). Complaints on sleep difficulties refer both to the duration of sleep, and to its quality (Knauth and Costa, 1996).

Differences in sleep patterns related to work systems were studied by Pilcher et al. (2000) by means of meta-analysis. The authors concluded that permanent night workers (those who always worked at night) were the ones with shorter sleep. Those results remit to the clinical evaluation of sleep performed by Walia et al. (2011), who observed that shift workers, particularly fixed shift workers, had greater difficulties with sleep onset. These data reveal the importance of considering shift work history when analyzing sleep symptom severity.

In a classical study comparing day workers, shift workers with rotating morning and afternoon shifts, and shift workers including night work, the more frequent complaints on sleep were related to shift systems that included night work, and also in the group of shift workers who later changed to day work (Knauth & Costa, 1996).

A debate in the relevant literature refers to possible long-term effects of night work on sleep, which would be reported after quitting night work. For some authors, there is no evidence that early experience with shift work results in later sleep difficulties (Webb, 1983; Niedhammer et al., 1994). Other authors show that transfer to day work does not guarantee a reduction in sleep-related disturbances (Dumont et al., 1987; 1997). In a recent study on this matter, Rotenberg et al. (2011) showed that difficulty maintaining sleep was more likely to be reported by former night workers regardless of the time devoted to night work in the past, and of how recently they had left night work.

4. Final remarks

This chapter has offered a description of prevalence and risk factors associated to insomnia. In fact, insomnia is related to socioeconomic and demographic characteristics, psychosocial causes, occupational factors, co-morbid medical disorders, abuse of alcohol and other aspects of lifestyle. The diversity of factors here described reveals the multifactorial nature of insomnia in terms of its etiology (Summers et al., 2006). The reciprocity between some factors contributes to the complexity of insomnia, as can be seen by the relationship between stress and sleep. In fact, stress impairs sleep quality, and disturbed sleep is likely to become a stressor in itself, thus promoting a vicious circle of stress and insomnia (Akerstedt, 2006). A better understanding of insomnia prevalence and incidence demands validated and consistent definitions and diagnostic criteria. Clearly, this will lead to a better data interpretation, thus enhancing our understanding of this important disorder.

5. References

Akerstedt, T.; Fredlund, P.; Gillberg, M. & Jansson, B. (2002b). Work load and work hours in relation to disturbed sleep and fatigue in a large representative sample, *Journal of Psychosomatic Research* Vol. 53 (N° 1): 585-588.

Akerstedt, T.; Knutsson, A.; Westerholm, P.; Theorell, T.; Alfredsson, L. & Kecklund, G. (2002a). Sleep disturbances, work stress and work hours: a cross-sectional study, *Journal of Psychosomatic Research* Vol. 53 (N° 3): 741-748.

Akerstedt, T. (2006). Psychosocial stress and impaired sleep, *Scandinavian Journal of Work, Environment & Health* Vol. 32 (N° 6, special issue): 493-501.

Akerstedt, T. (2003). Shift work and disturbed sleep/wakefulness, *Occupational Medicine (London)* Vol. 53 (N° 2): 89-94.

American Academy of Sleep Medicine. (2005). *The International Classification of Sleep Disorders, Second Edition (ICSD-2): Diagnostic and Coding Manual. Second Edition.*

American Psychiatric Association. (2000). *Diagnostic and Statistical Manual of Mental Disorders (DSM-IVTR). Fourth Edition, Text Revision.* Washington, DC: American Psychiatric Association.

American Sleep Disorders Association (ASDA). (1990). *International Classification of Sleep Disorders: Diagnostic and Coding Manual (ICSD).* Diagnostic Classification Steering Committee, Thorpy Mj, Chairman. Rochester, MN.

Ancoli-Israel, S. I. & Roth, T. (1999). Characteristics of insomnia in the United States: Result of the 1991 National Sleep Foundation Survey I, *Sleep* Vol. 22 (N° 2): 347-353.

Basta, M.; Chrousos, G. P.; Vela-Bueno, A. & Vgontzas, A. N. (2007). Chronic insomnia and stress system, *Sleep Medicine Clinics* June Vol. 2 (N° 2): 279–291.

Benca, R. M.; Ancoli-Israel, S. & Moldofsky, H. (2004). Special considerations in insomnia diagnosis and management: depressed, elderly, and chronic pain populations, *Journal of Clinical Psychiatry* Vol. 65 (Suppl 8): 26–35.

Bixler, E. O.; Vgontzas, A. N.; Lin, H. M.; Vela-Bueno, A. & Kales, A. (2002). Insomnia in Central Pennsylvania, *Journal of Psychosomatic Research* Vol. 53: 589-592.

Bixler, E. O.; Kales, A.; Soldatos, C. R.; Kales, J. D. & Healey, S. (1979). Prevalence of sleep disorders in the Los Angeles metropolitan area, *American Journal of Psychiatry* Vol. 136: 1257-1262.

Breslau, N.; Roth, T.; Rosenthal, L. & Andreski, P. (1996). Sleep disturbance and psychiatric disorders: A longitudinal epidemiological study of young adults, *Biological Psychiatry* Vol. 39: 411-418.

Brower, K. J.; Aldrich, M. S.; Robinson, E. A. R.; Zucker, R. A. & Greden, J. F. (2001). Insomnia, self medication, and relapse to alcoholism, *American Journal of Psychiatry* Vol. 158: 399–404.

Buysse, D. J. (2004). Insomnia, depression and aging. Assessing sleep and mood interactions in older adults, *Geriatrics* Vol. 59 (N° 2): 47-51.

Campos, H. H.; Bittencourt, L. R. A.; Haidar, M. A.; Tufik, S. & Baracat, E. C. (2005). Sleep disturbance prevalence in postmenopausal women, *Revista Brasileira de Ginecologia e Obstetrícia* Vol. 27 (N° 12): 731-736.

Coleman, R. M.; Roffwarg, H. P.; Kennedy, S. J.; Guilleminault, C.; Cinque, J.; Cohn, M. A.; Karacan, I.; Kupfer, D. J.; Lemmi, H.; Miles, L. E.; Orr, W. C.; Phillips, E. R.; Roth, T.; Sassin, J. F.; Schmidt, H. S.; Weitzman, E. D. & Dement, W. C. (1982). Sleep-wake disorders based on a polysomnographic diagnosis. A national cooperative study, *Journal of the American Medical Association* Vol. 247: 997-1003.

Dennerstein, L.; Dudley, L. E.; Hopper, J. L.; Guthrie, J. R. & Burger, H. G. (2000). A Prospective Population-Based Study of Menopausal Symptoms, *Obstetrics & Gynecology* Vol. 96 (Nº 3): 351-358.

Doghramji, K. (2006). The Epidemiology and Diagnosis of Insomnia, *The American Journal of Managed Care* S214-S220.

Dumont, M.; Montpaisir, J.; Infant-Rivard, C. (1987). Past experience of nightwork and present quality of life, *Sleep Research* Vol. 16: 40.

Dumont, M.; Montpaisir, J. & Infant-Rivard, C. (1997). Sleep Quality of Former Night-shift Workers, *International Journal of Occupational and Environmental Health* S10-S14.

Fahlén, G.; Knutsson, A.; Peter, R.; Akerstedt, T.; Nordin, M.; Alfredsson, L. & Westerholm, P. (2006). Effort-reward imbalance, sleep disturbances and fatigue, *International Archives of Occupational and Environmental Health Vol.* 79 (Nº 5): 371-378.

Foley, D. J.; Monjan, A. A.; Izmirlian, G.; Hays, J. C. & Blazer, D. G. (1999). Incidence and remission of insomnia among elderly adults in a biracial cohort, *Sleep* Vol. 22 (suppl. 2): S373-S378

Ford, D. E. & Kamerow, D. B. (1989). Epidemiologic study of sleep disturbances and psychiatric disorders. An opportunity for prevention?, *Journal of the American Medical Association* Vol. 262: 1479–1484.

Foster, J. H.; Marshall, E. J. & Peters, T. J. (2000). Application of a quality of life measure, the life situation survey (LSS) to alcohol-dependent subjects in relapse and remission, *Alcoholism: Clinical & Experimental Research* Vol. 24: 1687–1692.

Goral, A.; Lipsitz, J. D. & Grossa, R. (2010). The relationship of chronic pain with and without comorbid psychiatric disorder to sleep disturbance and health care utilization: Results from the Israel National Health Survey, *Journal of Psychosomatic Research* Vol. 69: 449–457.

Gupta, A.; Silman, A. J.; Ray, D.; Morriss, R.; Dickens, C.; MacFarlane, G. J.; Chiu, Y. H.; Nicholl, B. & McBeth, J. (2007). The role of psychosocial factors in predicting the onset of chronic widespread pain: results from a prospective population-based study, *Rheumatology (Oxford)* Vol.46: 666–71.

Gureje, O. (2007). Psychiatric aspects of pain, *Current Opinion in Psychiatry* Vol.20: 42–6.

Härmä, M.; Tenkanen, L.; Sjöblom, T.; Alikoski, T. & Heinsalmi, P. (1998) Combined effects of shift work and life-style on the prevalence of insomnia, sleep deprivation and daytime sleepiness, *Scandinavian Journal of Work, Environment & Health* Vol. 24 (Nº 4): 300-307.

Hausser, J.A., Mojzisch, A., Niesel, M., & Schulz-Hardt, S. (2010). Ten years on: A review of recent research on the Job Demand-Control (Support) Model and psychological wellbeing, *Work & Stress* Vol.24: 1-35.

Healey, E. S.; Kales, A.; Monroe, L. J.; Bixler, E. O.; Chamberlin, K. & Soldatos, C. R. (1981). Onset of insomnia: role of life-stress events, *Psychosomatic Medicine* Vol. 43 (Nº 5): 439-451.

Ingre, M. & Akerstedt, T. (2004). Effect of accumulated night work during the working lifetime, on subjective health and sleep in monozygotic twins, *Journal of Sleep Research* Vol. 13 (Nº 1): 45-8.

Janson, C.; Gislason, T.; De Backer, W.; Plaschke, P.; Björnsson, E.; Hetta, J.; Kristbjarnason, H.; Vermeire, P. & Boman, G. (1995). Prevalence of sleep disturbances among young adults in three European countries, *Sleep* Vol. 18 (N° 7): 589-97.

Johnson, E. O. & Breslau, N. (2001) Sleep problems and substance use in adolescence. *Drug and Alcohol Dependence* Vol. 64 (N° 1): 1-7.

Johnson, J.V., & Hall, E.M. (1988). Job strain, workplace social support and cardiovascular disease: A cross-sectional study of a random sample of the Swedish working population, *American Journal of Public Health* Vol. 78 (N° 10): 1336-1342.

Kalimo, R.; Tenkanen, L.; Härmä, M.; Poppius, E. & Heinsalmi, P. (2000). Job stress and sleep disorders: Findings from the Helsinki Heart Study, *Stress Medicine* Vol. 16 (N° 2): 65–75.

Kalleinen, N. (2008). Sleep and menopause - hormone therapy and sleep deprivation [Tese]. Turku, Finland: University of Turku.

Karasek, R. A. (1979). Job demands, job decision latitude, and mental strain: Implications for job redesign, *Administrative Science Quarterly* Vol. 24 (N° 2): 285-307.

Karasek, R., & Theorell, T. (1990). *Healthy work: Stress, productivity and the reconstruction of working life.* New York: Basic Books

Kim, H. C.; Kim, B. K.; Min, K. B.; Min, J. Y.; Hwang, S. H. & Park, S. G. (2011). Association between job stress and insomnia in Korean workers. *Journal of Occupational Health* Vol. 53: 164-174.

Kim, K.; Uchiyama, M.; Okawa, M.; Liu, X. & Ogihara, R. (2000). Na epidemiological study of insomnia among the Japanese general population, *Sleep* Vol. 23 (N° 1): 1-7.

Knauth, P. & Costa, G. (1996). Psychosocial Effects. In: *Shiftwork. Problems and Solutions.* Colquhoun, W. P.; Costa, G.; Folkard, S. & Knauth, P. (orgs). Berlin: Peter Lang, p. 89-112.

Krystal, A. D. (2003). Insomnia in women, Clinical Cornestone Vol. 5 (N° 3): 41-50.

Kudielka, B. M.; Von Känel, R.; Gander, M. L. & Fischer, J. E. (2004). Effort-reward imbalance, overcommitment and sleep in a working population, *Work and Stress* Vol. 18 (N° 2): 167-178.

Kuppermann, M.; Lubeck, D. P.; Mazonson, P. D.; Patrick, D. L.; Stewart, A. L.; Buesching, D. P. & Fifer, S. K. (1995). Sleep problems and their correlates in a working population, *Journal of General Internal Medicine* Vol. 10: 25–32.

Landis, C. A. & Moe, K. E. (2004). Sleep and menopause, *The Nursing Clinics of North America* Vol. 39: 97-115.

Lamberg, L. (2003). Illness not age itself most often the trigger of sleep problems in older adults, *Journal of the American Medical Association* Vol. 290 (N° 3): 319-323.

Lautenbacher, S.; Kundermann, B. & Krieg, J. C. (2006). Sleep deprivation and pain perception, *Sleep Medicine Reviews* Vol. 10: 357–69.

LeBlanc, M.; Mérette, C.; Savard, J.; Ivers, H.; Baillargeon, L. & Morin, C. M. (2009). Incidence and risk factors of insomnia in a population-based sample, *Sleep* Vol. 32 (N° 8): 1027-1037.

Lee, K. A.; Baker, F. C.; Newton, K. M. & Ancoli-Israel, S. (2008). The influence of reproductive status and age on women's sleep, *Journal of Womens's Health* Vol. 17 (N° 7): 1209-1214.

Léger, D.; Guilleminault, C.; Dreyfus, J. P.; Delahaye, C. & Paillard, M. (2000). Prevalence of insomnia in a survey of 12778 adults in France, *Journal of Sleep Research* Vol. 9: 35-42.

Li, R. H. Y.; Ho, S. C. & Fong, S. Y. Y. (2002). Gender differences in insomnia - a study in the Hong Kong Chinese population, *Journal of Psychosomatic Research* Vol. 53: 601-609.

Lustberg, L. & Reynolds, C. F. (2000). Depression and insomnia: questions of cause and effect, *Sleep Medicine Reviews* Vol. 4 (N° 3): 253-262.

Maartens, L. W.; Leusink, G. L.; Knottnerus, J. A.; Smeets, C. G. & Pop, V. J. (2001). Climacteric complaints in the community, *Family Practice - an International Journal* Vol. 18 (N° 2): 189-194.

McCracken, L. M. & Iverson, G. L. (2002). Disrupted sleep patterns and daily functioning in patients with chronic pain, *Pain Research & Management* Vol. 7: 75–9.

Mahfoud, Y.; Talih, F.; Streem, D. & Budur K. (2009). Sleep Disorders in Substance Abusers: How Common Are They?, *Psychiatry* Vol. 6 (N° 9): 38–42

Mai, E. & Buysse, D. J. (2008). Insomnia: Prevalence, Impact, Pathogenesis, Differential Diagnosis, and Evaluation, *Sleep Medicine Clinics* Vol. 3 (N° 2): 167–174.

Marchi, N. S. A.; Reimão, R.; Tognola, W. A. & Cordeiro, Jj. A. (2004). Analysis of the prevalence of insomnia in the adult population of São José do Rio Preto, Brazil, *Arquivos de Neuropsiquiatria* Vol. 62 (N° 3-B): 764-768.

Martikainen, K.; Partinen, M.; Hasan, J.; Laippala, P.; Urponen, H. & Vuori, I. (2003). The impact of somatic health problems on insomnia in middle age, *Sleep Medicine* Vol. 4 (N° 3): 201-6.

Moffitt, P. F.; Kalucy, E. C.; Kalucy, R.S.; Baum, F. E. & Cooke, R. D. (1991). Sleep difficulties, pain and other correlates, *Journal of Internal Medicine* 1991; Vol. 230 (N° 3): 245-249.

Montplaisir, J.; Lorrain, J.; Denesle, R. & Petit, D. (2001). Sleep in menopause: Differential effects of two forms of hormone replacement therapy, *Menopause* Vol. 8: 10-16.

Morin, C. M.; Leblanc. M.; Daley, M.; Gregoire, J. P. & Mérette, C. (2006). Epidemiology of insomnia: prevalence, self-help treatments, consultations, and determinants of help-seeking behaviors, *Sleep Medicine* Vol. 7: 123-130.

Nakata, A.; Haratani, T.; Takahashi, M.; Kawakami, N.; Arito, H.; Fujioka, Y.; Shimizu, H.; Kobayashi, F. & Araki, S. (2001). Job stress, social support at work, and insomnia in Japanese shift workers. *Journal of Human Ergology (Tokyo)*. Dec Vol. 30 (N° 1-2): 203-209.

National-sleep-foundation. (2005). Sleep in America poll 2005. In: http://www.sleepfoundation.org/_content/hottopics/2005_summary_of_findings.pdf. Accessed in September, 2005.

Niedhammer, I.; Left, F. & Marne, M. J. (1994). Effects of shift work on sleep among French nurses: A longitudinal study. *Journal of Occupational Medicine*, Vol. 36 (N° 6): 667-674.

Nomura, K.; Nakao, M.; Takeuchi, T. & Yano, E. (2009). Associations of insomnia with job strain, control, and support among male Japanese workers, *Sleep Medicine* Vol. 10: 626-629.

Ohayon, M. M. (2002). Epidemiology of insomnia: what we know and what we still need to learn, *Sleep Medicine* Vol. 6 (N° 2): 97-111.

Ohayon, M. M. & Bader, G. (2010). Prevalence and correlates of insomnia in the Swedish population aged 19–75 years, *Sleep Medicine* Vol. 11: 980–986.

Ohayon, M. M.; Caulet, M.; Priest, R. G. & Guilleminault, C. (1997). DSM-IX and ICSD-90 insomnia symptoms and sleep dissatisfaction, *The British Journal of Psychiatry* Vol. 171 (N° 10): 382-388.

Ohayon, M. M. & Hong, S. C. (2002). Prevalence of insomnia and associated factors in South Korea, *Journal of Psychosomatic Research* Vol. 53: 593-600.

Ohayon, M. M. & Partinen, M. (2002). Insomnia and global sleep dissatisfaction in Finland, *Journal of Sleep Research* Vol. 11: 339-346.

Ohayon, M. M. & Roth, T. (2001) What are the contributing factors for insomnia in the general population? *Journal of Psychosomatic Research* Vol. 51: 745-755.

Ohayon, M. M. & Roth, T. (2003). Place of chronic insomnia in the course of depressive and anxiety disorders, *Journal of Psychiatric Research* Vol. 37 (N° 1): 9-15.

Ohayon, M. M. & Zulley, J. (2001). Correlates of global sep dissatisfaction in the German population. *Sleep* Vol. 24 (N° 7): 780-787.

Ota, A.; Masue, T.; Yasuda, N.; Tsutsumi, A.; Mino, Y. & Ohara, H. (2005). Association between psychosocial job characteristics and insomnia: an investigation using two relevant job stress models—the demand-control-support (DCS) model and the effort-reward imbalance (ERI) model, *Sleep Medicine* Vol. 6: 353-358.

Ota, A.; Masue, T.; Yasuda, N.; Tsutsumi, A.; Mino, Y. & Ohara, H. (2009). Psychosocial job characteristics and insomnia: A prospective cohort study using the Demand-Control-Support (DCS) and Effort–Reward Imbalance (ERI) job stress models, *Sleep Medicine* Vol. 10: 1112-1117.

Pallensen, S.; Nordhus, I. H.; Nielsen, H.; Havik, O. E; Kvale, G.; Johnsen, B. H. & Skjotskift, S. (2001). Prevalence of insomnia in the adult Norwegian population, *Sleep* Vol. 24 (N° 7): 771-779.

Panda-Moreno, M.; Beltrám, C. A.; Aldrete, M. E. A.; Roal, P. L. M. & Estrada, J. G. S. (2001). Prevalence of sleep disorders in the elderly, *Caderno de Saúde Pública* Vol. 17 (N°1): 63-69.

Pedro, A. O.; Pinto-Neto, A. M.; Costa-Paiva, L. H. S.; Osis, M. J. D. & Hardy, E. E. (2003). Climacteric syndrome: a population-based study in Campinas, SP, Brazil, *Revista de Saúde Pública* Vol. 37 (N° 6): 735-742

Pérez, J. A. M.; Garcia, F. C.; Palacios, S. (2009). Pérez, M. Epidemiology of risk factors and symptoms associated with menopause in Spanish women, *Maturitas* Vol. 62: 30-36.

Peter, R.; Geissler, H. & Siegrist, J. (1998). Associations of effort-reward imbalance at work and reported symptoms in different groups of male and female public transport workers, *Stress Medicine* Vol. 14: 175–182

Peter, R. & Siegrist, J. (2000). Psychosocial work environment and the risk of coronary heart disease, *International Archives of Occupational and Environmental Health* Vol. 73: S4-S45.

Phillips, B. A.; Collop, N. A.; Drake, C.; Consens, F.; Vgontzas, A. N. & Weaver, T. E. (2008) Sleep disorders and medical conditions in women, *Journal of Women's Health* Vol. 17 (N° 7): 1191-1199.

Phillips, B. A. & Danner, F. J. (1995) Cigarette smoking and sleep disturbance, *Archives of Internal Medicine* Vol. 155 (N° 7): 734-737.

Pilcher, J. J.; Lambert, B. J. & Huffcutt, A. I. (2000). Differential effects of permanent and rotating shifts on self-report sleep length: a meta-analytic review, *Sleep* Vol. 23 (N° 2): 155-163.

Pires, M. L.; Benedito-Silva, A. A.; Mello, M. T.; Pompeia Sdel, G. & Tufik, S. (2007) Sleep habits and complaints of adults in the city of São Paulo, Brazil, in 1987 and 1995. *Brazilian Journal of Medical and Biological Research* Vol. 40 (N° 11): 1505-1515.

Polo-Kantola, P.; Erkkola, R.; Helenius, H.; Irjala, K. & Polo, O. (1998). When does estrogen replacement therapy improve sleep quality, American Journal of Obstetrics and Gynecology Vol. 178: 1002-1009.

Presser, H. B. (2003). *Working in a 24/7 Economy: Challenges for American Families.* NY: Russel Sage Foundation

Purdie, D.; Empson, J.; Crichton, C. & Macdonald, L. (1995) Hormone replacement therapy, sleep quality and psychological wellbeing, *British Journal of Obstetrics and Gynaecology* Vol. 102: 735-739.

Qureshi, A. & Lee-Chiong, T. Jr. (2004) Medications and their effects on sleep, *Medical Clinics of North America* Vol. 88 (N° 3): 751-766.

Ramakrishnan, K. & Scheid, D. C. (2007). Treatment Options for Insomnia, *American Family Physician* Vol. 76 (N° 4): 517-526.

Ribet, C. & Derriennic, F. (1999). Age, working conditions, and sleep disorders: a longitudinal analysis in the French cohort E.S.T.E.V., *Sleep* Vol. 22 (N° 4): 491-504.

Robaina, J. R.; Lopes, C. S.; Rotenberg, L.; Faerstein, E.; Fischer, F. M.; Moreno, C. R. C.; Werneck, G. L. & Chor, D. (2009). Stressful life events and insomnia complaints among nursing assistants from a university hospital in Rio de Janeiro: The Pro-Saude Study, *Revista Brasileira de Epidemiologia* Vol. 12 (N° 3): 501-509.

Roberts, R. E.; Shema, S. J.; Kaplan, G. A. & Strawbridge, W. J. (2000). Sleep Complaints and Depression in an Aging Cohort: A Prospective Perspective, *American Journal of Psychiatry* Vol. 157: 81–88.

Rocha, F. L.; Guerra, H. L. & Costa, M. F. F. L. (2002). Prevalence of insomnia and associated socio-demographic factors in a Brazilian community: the Bambuí study, *Sleep Medicine* Vol. 3: 121-126.

Rotenberg, L.; Griep, R. H.; Silva-Costa, A. & Diniz, T. B. (2011). Long-term deleterious effects of night work on sleep, *Sleep Science*, 2011 (in press)

Roth, T. (2001). New developments for treating sleep disorders, *Journal of Clinical Psychiatry* Vol. 62 (suppl 10): 3-4.

Roth, T.; Coulouvrat, C.; Hajak, G.; Lakoma, M. D.; Sampson, N. A.; Shahly, V.; Shillington, A. C.; Stephenson, J. J.; Walsh, J. K. & Kessler, R. C. (2011). Prevalence and perceived health associated with insomnia based on DSM-IV-TR; International Statistical Classification of Diseases and Related Health Problems, Tenth Revision; and Research Diagnostic Criteria/International Classification of Sleep Disorders, Second Edition criteria: results from the America Insomnia Survey, *Biological Psychiatry* Mar 15; Vol. 69 (N° 6): 592-600.

Roth, T.; Krystal, A. D. & Lieberman, J. A. (2007). Long-term issues in the treatment of sleep disorders. *CNS Spectrums* Vol. 12 (N° 7 Suppl 10): 1–14.

Roth, T. & Roehrs, T. (2003). Insomnia: epidemiology, characteristics, and consequences. *Clinical Cornerstone* Vol. 5 (N° 3): 5-15.

Rugulies, R.; Norborg, M.; Sørensen, T. S.; Knudsen, L. E. & Burr, H. (2009). Effort-reward imbalance at work and risk of sleep disturbances. Cross-sectional and prospective results from the Danish Work Environment Cohort Study, *Journal of Psychosomatic Research* Vol. 66 (N° 1): 75-83.

Saletu-Zyhlarz, G.; Anderer, P.; Gruber, G.; Mandl, M.; Gruber, D.; Metka, M.; Huber, J.; Oettel, M.; Graser, T.; Abu-bakr, M. H.; Gratzhofer, E. & Saletu, B. (2003). Insomnia related to postmenopausal syndrome and hormone replacement therapy: Sleep laboratory studies on baseline differences between patients and controls and double-blind, placebo-controlled investigations on the effects of a novel estrogen-progestogen combination (Climodien, Lafamme) versus estrogen alone, *Journal of Sleep Research* Vol. 12: 239-254.

Sarti, C. D.; Chiantera, A.; Graziottin, A.; Ognisanti, F.; Sidoli, C.; Mincigrucci, M.; Parazzini, F. & Gruppo Di Studio Iper, Aogoi, (2005). Hormone therapy and sleep quality in women around menopause, Menopause Vol. 12: 545-551.

Schnall, P.; Belkić, K.; Landsbergis, P. & Baker, D. (2000). Why the workplace and cardiovascular disease? In: *The workplace and cardiovascular disease. Occupational medicine: states-of-art reviews*, Schnall, P.; Belkic, K.; Landsbergis, P. A.; et al, Editors, Hanley and Belfus. Philadelphia, pp 1-5.

Shaver, J. L. & Zenk, S. N. (2000). Sleep disturbance in menopause, *Journal of Women's Health and Gender-Based Medicine* Vol. 9 (N° 2): 109-118.

Shin, C.; Lee, S.; Lee, T.; Shin, K.; Yi, H.; Kim, K. & Cho, N. (2005). Prevalence of insomnia and its relationship to menopausal status in middle-aged Korean women. *Psychiatry and Clinical Neuroscience* Vol. 59: 395–402.

Siegrist, J. (1996). Adverse health effects of high effort - low reward conditions at work. *Journal of Occupational and Health Psychology* Vol. 1: 27-43.

Simon, G. E. & Von Korff, M. (1997). Prevalence, burden, and treatment of insomnia in primary care. *American Journal of Psychiatry* Vol. 154: 1417–1423.

Souza, C. L.; Aldrighi, J. M. & Lorenzi Filho, G. (2005). Quality of sleep of climacteric women in São Paulo: some significant aspects, *Revista da Associação Médica Brasileira* Vol. 51 (N° 3): 170-176.

Summers, M. O.; Crisostomo, M. I. & Stepanski, E. J. (2006). Recent developments in the classification, evaluation, and treatment of insomnia, *Chest* Vol. 130: 276 –286.

Sutton, D. A.; Moldofsky, H. & Badley, E. M. (2001). Insomnia and health problems in Canadians, *Sleep* Vol. 24 (N° 6): 665-670.

Tjepkema, M. (2005). Insomnia. *Health Reports* Vol. 17 (N° 1): 9-25.

Üstun, T. B.; Privett, M.; Lecrubier, Y.; Weiller, E.; Simon, G.; Korten, A.; Bassett, S. S.; Maier, W.; Sartorius, N. (1996). Form, frequency and burden of sleep problems in general health care: a report from the WHO collaborative study on psychological problems in general health care, *European Psychiatry* Vol. 11 (N° 1): S5-S10.

Vela-Bueno, A.; Iceta, M. & Fernández, C. (1999). Prevalencia de los trastornos del sueño en la ciudad de Madrid, *Gaceta Sanitaria* Vol. 13 (N° 6): 441-448.

Walia, H. K.; Hayes, A. L.; Przepyszny, K. A.; Karumanchi, P. & Patel, S. R. (2011) Clinical presentation of shift workers to a sleep clinic, Sleep Breath [Epub ahead of print]

Webb, W. B. (1983). Are there permanent effects of night shift work on sleep? *Biological Psychology* Vol. 16: 273-283.

Wilson, K. G.; Eriksson, M. Y.; D'Eon, J. L.; Mikail, S. F. & Emery, P. C. (2002). Major depression and insomnia in chronic pain, *The Clinical Journal of Pain* Vol. 18: 77–83.

Wong, W. S. & Fielding, R. (2011). Prevalence of insomnia among Chinese adults in Hong Kong: a population-based study. *Journal of Sleep Research* Vol. 20: 117–126.

World Health Organization. The ICD-10 classification of mental and behavioural disorders. (1992). Clinical descriptions and diagnostic guidelines. Geneva: World Health Organization.

Yaniv, G. (2004). Insomnia, biological clock, and the bedtime decision: an economic perspective, *Health Economics* Vol. 13: 1-8.

Young, T. B. (2005). Natural history of chronic insomnia. NIH Insomnia abstract. *Journal of Clinical Sleep Medicine* Vol. 1 (suppl): e466-e467.

Zhang, B. & Wing, Y. K. (2006). Sex differences in insomnia: A metaanalysis, *Sleep* Vol. 29: 85.

2

Drugs Inducing Insomnia as an Adverse Effect

Ntambwe Malangu
University of Limpopo, Medunsa Campus, School of Public Health, South Africa

1. Introduction

Insomnia is a symptom, not a stand-alone disease. By definition, insomnia is "difficulty initiating or maintaining sleep, or both" or the perception of poor quality sleep (APA, 1994). As an adverse effect of medicines, it has been documented for several drugs. This chapter describes some drugs whose safety profile includes insomnia. In doing so, it discusses the mechanisms through which drug-induced insomnia occurs, the risk factors associated with its occurrence, and ends with some guidance on strategies to prevent and manage drug-induced insomnia.

2. How drugs induce insomnia

There are several mechanisms involved in the induction of insomnia by drugs. Some drugs affects sleep negatively when being used, while others affect sleep and lead to insomnia when they are withdrawn. Drugs belonging to the first category include anticonvulsants, some antidepressants, steroids and central nervous stimulant drugs such amphetamine and caffeine. With regard to caffeine, the mechanism by which caffeine is able to promote wakefulness and insomnia has not been fully elucidated (Lieberman, 1992). However, it seems that, at the levels reached during normal consumption, caffeine exerts its action through antagonism of central adenosine receptors; thereby, it reduces physiologic sleepiness and enhances vigilance (Benington et al., 1993; Walsh et al., 1990; Rosenthal et al., 1991; Bonnet and Arand, 1994; Lorist et al., 1994). In contrast to caffeine, methamphetamine and methylphenidate produce wakefulness by increasing dopaminergic and noradrenergic neurotransmission (Gillman and Goodman, 1985). With regard to withdrawal, it may occur in 40% to 100% of patients treated chronically with benzodiazepines, and can persist for days or weeks following discontinuation. Withdrawal symptoms include dizziness, confusion, and depression (Lader et al., 2009).

Another feature of discontinuation of drugs is rebound insomnia, which is an increase in insomnia symptoms beyond their baseline level. Rebound is thought to be associated primarily with short-acting benzodiazepines. Patients who demonstrate rebound insomnia tend to have worse baseline sleep and higher medication doses than patients without rebound (Merlotti et al., 1991; Roehrs et al., 1986; Hajak et al., 1998; Griffiths and Weerts, 1997). While insomnia can also result from chronic use of hypnotics such as benzodiazepines and other sedatives, the following classes of drugs can cause insomnia when withdrawn: central nervous depressants such as alcohol, certain antidepressants, and barbiturates, opioids both legal and illicit such as cocaine, heroin, marijuana; as well as monoamine oxidase inhibitors and phencyclidine.

Moreover, it is known that adrenal dysfunction can cause catecholamine secretion that may lead to sympathetic activation and insomnia. Similarly, excessive glucocorticoid levels also cause insomnia (Attarian, 2004). Furthermore, an indirect effect through neurologic and psychiatric effects such as headaches, irritability, anxiety and agitation may also lead to insomnia. This is the case for commonly prescribed hypnotics that cause irritability and many psychoactive drugs that induce abnormal movements during sleep (Zammit et al., 1999; Breslau et al., 1996). Drugs which suppress rapid eye movement (REM), commonly result in REM rebound nightmares on withdrawal, as in the case of opioid analgesics. While such drugs are being taken, the relative lack of REM sleep may lead to underestimation of the severity of sleep apnea. Drugs which suppress slow-wave sleep (SWS) commonly leave the patient unrested, as seen with corticosteroids.

Parasomnias, defined as unusual behaviours during sleep such as sleepwalking, sleep-talking, teeth grinding, bedwetting, sleep starts, sleep terrors, and confusion awakenings are sleep disturbances associated and leading to drug-induced insomnia. Sleepwalking may occur in over 15% of healthy children and 3% of adults, typically take place during short wave sleep. Several medications which increase this stage of sleep may induce sleep-walking: lithium, thioridazine, and amitriptyline. Drugs that suppress REM sleep increase the likelihood of some parasomnias: tricyclic antidepressants, for example, and triazolam. Nightmares, reported at least occasionally by 40-50% of adults, are known to be associated with REM sleep (Novak and Shapiro, 1997).

Drugs which predispose to nightmares include beta-blockers, especially those that more easily penetrate into the brain, like propranolol. Stimulant drugs which disrupt night-time sleep include theophylline and sympathomimetic bronchodilators such as ephedrine. Drugs which may worsen sleep apnea include alcohol, opioid analgesics, and anaesthetic drugs. Among the cardiovascular drugs, some antihypertensive drugs are particularly important in their effects on sleep, generally a decrease in the duration of REM sleep, but it is unclear how significant these effects are for patients. REM sleep is decreased by blockers of beta-adrenoreceptors like pindolol, stimulants of alpha adrenoreceptors like clonidine and guanfacine, serotonin stimulators like ritanserin and ketanserin, and methyldopa. Only reserpine increases REM sleep. Beta-blockers like propranolol in particular increase wakefulness by causing insomnia and nightmares, and by suppressing REM sleep. However, the frequency of these effects may be low, especially with types of beta-blockers that do not readily penetrate to the brain, like atenolol (Novak and Shapiro, 1997; Roehrs et al., 2000; Roth and Roehrs, 2003).

Other drugs produce insomnia by interfering with melatonin. Melatonin has the ability to influence the timing of the circadian sleep-wake cycle (Sack et al., 2000), has sedative effects possibly via direct inhibition of the suprachiasmatic nucleus via a feedback loop (Dubocovitch, 1995). It is suggested that melatonin promotes sleep in humans, presumably by inhibiting circadian wakefulness mechanisms and affecting the activity of brain networks compatible with sleep induction (Cajochen et al., 2003; Wyatt et al., 200; Liu et al., 1997; Shocaht et al., 1997; Gorfine et al., 2006). However, numerous studies have shown decreased melatonin levels in the elderly relative to subjects aged less than 30 years (Sharma et al,

1989; Zhou et al., 2003) because of the decline in the number of pinealocytes, and/or neuronal degeneration and resultant circadian desynchrony (Kripke et al., 1998). Yet, melatonin deficiency many be induced by a variety of medications commonly used by the elderly, including beta-blockers and non-steroidal anti-inflammatory drugs (Gorfine et al., 2006; Liu et al., 1997).

Examples of classes of drugs inducing insomnia and their mechanisms of action

Through melatonin

- Beta-blockers
- Non-steroidal anti-inflammatory drugs

Through interfering with REM

- Beta-blockers
- Tricyclic antidepressants: eg.
- Stimulant drugs : eg. Theophylline
- Serotonin stimulators: eg. ritanserin

Through interfering with slow-wave sleep

- Corticosteroids

Through increasing dopaminergic and noradrenergic neurotransmission

- methamphetamine
- methylphenidate

Through withdrawal

- Benzodiazepines
- Barbiturates
- Opioids such as cocaine, heroin, marijuana

Through direct action by antagonism of central adenosine receptors

- Caffeine

Box 1. Mechanisms involved in drug induction of insomnia

3. Risk factors of drug-induced insomnia

From the mechanisms of action described above, it is appears that several factors would contribute to the occurrence of insomnia as a result of using a particular drug or withdrawing it. Reports of sleep disturbances associated with therapeutic drugs appeared in the 1970s and 1980s. Nightmares were observed with the initiation or withdrawal of tricyclic antidepressants and with the use of neuroleptic drugs (Strayhorn and Nash, 1978). Although levodopa was introduced in the 1960s, reports of levodopa-induced sleep disruptions did not appear until several years later (Sharf et al 1978).

Factors related to a particular drug include the chemical structure of the drug that dictates its activities, its pharmacological mechanisms of action, and the dosage used in a particular patient (Lancel, 1999; Mendelson et al., 1983; Olsen and Tobin, 1990). As shown below some drugs induce insomnia only when a certain level of dosage is reached. Factors related to an individual patient include race, lower socioeconomic status, and unemployment as well as age, sex, use of medications and comorbidities.

Several studies suggest there are ethnic and racial differences in sleep disturbances. Studies exploring associations between disturbed sleep and health-related quality of life (HR-QOL) have examined the role of comorbid conditions, gender, and race/ethnicity (Krystal, 2007; Baldwin et al., 2004; Katz and McHorney, 2002; Chowdhury et al., 2008). As with studies of sleep disturbances, the majority of HR-QOL research focused on differences between African American and Caucasian participants. Elderly African Americans with mild sleep apnea had significantly poorer physical and mental HRQOL than African Americans without it (Redline et al., 1997; Stepnowsky et al., 2000). African American, Hispanic, and other minority participants had both worse quality of sleep and poorer well-being than Caucasian participants (Jean-Louis et al., 2000). However, when sex, education, age, marital status, and healthcare coverage were controlled for, Caucasians were more likely to report not getting enough sleep than African Americans and Hispanics; when mood, medication use, socioeconomic status and perceived health were controlled for, Caucasians reported more restless sleep than African Americans (Kutner et al., 2004).

With regard to age, as explained above, the extent of melatonin suppression may be more profound in the elderly than in younger subjects. In addition to medications, a variety of primary conditions, such as chronic pain, myocardial infarction, and ischemic stroke are strongly associated with decreased melatonin levels in the elderly as animal studies have shown decreased levels of the Mel1a receptor with aging (Garfinkel et al., 1995; Murphy et al., 1996; Van den Heuven et al., 1997; Richardson and Tate, 2000). The elderly constitutes a group of individuals who are known as more susceptible to actions of drugs such as antidepressants, antihistaminic drugs, certain antipsychotics, and amphetamines (Fick et al., 2003). Furthermore, people who are elderly have a higher incidence of general medical conditions and are more likely to be taking medications that cause sleep disruption. Sleep studies objectively confirm the disturbed sleep of asthmatics. They are often woken with coughing, wheezing, and breathlessness. Similar problems apply to patients with chronic obstructive pulmonary disease (COPD or emphysema). Besides direct drug effects on their sleep, asthmatics suffer many other factors affecting sleep, such as gastroesophageal reflux, which can be aggravated by theophylline. Theophylline also has a central nervous system stimulatory effect that can disturb sleep, particularly in patients newly taking this drug.

With regard to commonly used medications, the following medicines are reported to promote chronic insomnia. These include selective serotonin reuptake inhibitors, lamotrigine, phenytoin, atorvastatin and oral contraceptives. Other risk factors of insomnia include the patient's health status, susceptibility, and co-morbidity (Balter and Uhlenhuth, 1992; Sharpley and Cowen, 1995;Espiritu, 2008; Saddichha, 2010).

With regard to comorbidities, the incidence of insomnia in hypertensive Japanese patients under antihypertensive therapy has been reported as 0.77/100 person-years; the factors contributing to insomnia onset were α blockers (OR, 2.38; 95% confidence interval [CI], 1.14-4.98), β blockers (OR, 1.54; 95% CI, 0.99-2.39), and calcium channel blockers (OR, 0.62; 95% CI, 0.43-0.90) compared with angiotensin-converting enzyme inhibitors; female sex (OR, 1.76; 95% CI, 1.27-2.44); complication of gastric/duodenal disorders (OR, 2.35; 95% CI, 1.14-4.86) or musculoskeletal system/connective tissue disorders (OR, 2.43; 95% CI, 1.23-4.79); and concomitant antihypertensive therapy (Tanabe et al., 2011). In patients suffering from myasthenia gravis, the prevalence of insomnia was 39.1% (Qui et al., 2010). Lastly, sleep disturbance is one of the most common complaints reported in 74-96% of patients suffering from Parkinson's disease. Insomnia is associated with increased morbidity and mortality caused by cardiovascular disease and psychiatric disorders and has other major public health and social consequences, such as accidents and absenteeism (Roth and Roehrs, 2003).

Risk factors associated with drug-induced insomnia

- Age
- Race and ethnicity
- Sex
- Medication use and drug interactions
- Comorbidities

Box 2. Risk factors for drug induced insomnia

4. Specific classes of drugs reported to cause insomnia

The following list is not comprehensive or exhaustive; it is purely presented for illustration purposes.

1. Amino-quinolones

Atovaquone plus proguanil, a combination that was used in the preventive and curative treatment of malaria has been reported to produce insomnia in 5.2% of patients (van Genderen et al., 2007).

2. Anabolic steroids

It is well known that the abuse of anabolic steroids can cause the stimulation of the nervous system and this may result in euphoria or and insomnia (Papazisis et al., 2007; Kanayama et al., 2008).

3. Anti-ADHD

Methylphenidate, a drug used to treat attention deficit hyperkinetic disorder (ADHD), was reported to produce insomnia in 19 of 62 patients who were included in an open label trial (Gucuyener et al., 2003).

4. Anti-asthmatic drugs

Insomnia was one of the common side effects in 84 patients who completed a randomized trial of albuterol/salbutamol (Kissel et al., 2001). Insomnia was also reported in 1.75% of the 110 participants with COPD in a trial involving theophylline (Zhou et al., 2006).

5. Antidepressants

In an open-label phase of a relapse prevention study, duloxetine (60 mg QD) was shown to be effective in the treatment of depression; among the 533 participants, insomnia was reported in over 10% of patients (Hudson et al., 2007).

6. Antiepileptic drugs

Lamotrigine led to insomnia in 2 of 29 patients treated for refractory epilepsy (Garcia-Escriva et al., 2004). Levetiracetam led to insomnia in 105 (7.5%) of 1422 patients observed during studies (Ben-Menachem et al., 2003; Mula et al., 2004). Insomnia was reported in 9% of patients who were treated with a median dose of 300mg per day of topiramate (Giannokodimos S et al., 2005)

7. Antihistamines

Insomnia has been reported in 30% taking loratadine plus pseudoephedrine versus 21% taking placebo (Berkowitz et al., 1989; Supiyaphun et al., 2002).

8. Anti-muscarinic drugs

In a meta-analysis of 72 original randomized trials of antimuscarinic drugs, namely, oxybutynin, tolterodine, fesoterodine, propiverine, solifenacin, darifenacin, and trospiu, adverse effects reported were, among others, insomnia and vertigo. The trials involved adults with overactive bladder using standard doses of medications (Paquette et al., 2011).

9. Anti-obesity drugs

Insomnia was one of the most common adverse effect of monoamine system drugs such as sibutramine, bupropion, and tesofensine (Nathan et al., 2010).

10. Antipsychotic drugs

Aripiprazole is known to produce fewer extrapyramidal effects, but in patients taking 15mg per day, insomnia in 42% of patients versus 18% in those taking the placebo (Shim et al., 2007; Carvajal et al., 2007).

In the 40-week extension of a clinical trial, insomnia was of the common adverse effects seen in over 10% of patients treated with asenapine (McIntyre et al., 2010).

11. Antiretroviral drugs

Efavirenz is known to produce neuropsychiatric effects including insomnia in up to 50% of patients (Kenedi and Goforth, 2011; Jena et al., 2009; Alavena et al., 2006). In a trial of single-pill fixed-dose regimen containing emtricitabine, tenofovir and efavirenz, four patients discontinued the trial because of insomnia (Airoldi et al., 2010). Insomnia has been reported in 5% to 16% patients on a regimen containing emtricitabine (Palacisos et al., 2008).

12. Anti-tuberculosis agents

Of the 18 patients identified with neuropsychiatric problems in 18 French patients, six had insomnia (Fekih et al., 2011).

13. Benzimidazoles

Albendazole, in a clinical trial of 168 patients, led to insomnia in 2 patients that have been treated for 7 days due to heavy infestation (Sirivichayakul et al., 2003).

14. Complementary and alternative medicines (CAM)

Despite its voluntary recall of Pai You Guo in 2009, clinicians have noted its continued use among Brazilian-born women in Massachusetts. The majority of users (85%) reported at least one side effect, among them insomnia in 26% of respondents (Cohen et al., 2011).

15. Cholinesterase inhibitors

Donepezil and galantamine have been reported to have induced insomnia in some patients (Kavirajan and Schneider, 2007).

16. Cox-2 inhibitors

Celecoxib and rofecoxib, of the 142 reports received by the Australian Adverse Reactions Advisory Committee (ADRAC), 21 cases were about insomnia (ADRAC, 2003). This neuropsychiatric reaction seems to be a class effect.

17. Fluoroquinolones

Drugs of this group such as gatifloxacin, gemifloxacin, and moxifloxacin produce mild central nervous complications including insomnia (Sable and Murakawa, 2003; Sable and Murakawa, 2004). Other psychiatric effects include headaches, and agitation that occurred in 2-4% of patients (Saravolatz and Leggett, 2003). In double-masked, randomized, comparative trials of sparfloxacin (a 400-mg oral loading dose followed by 200 mg/d for 10 days) versus standard therapies (erythromycin, cefaclor, ofloxacin, clarithromycin, and ciprofloxacin), insomnia was reported in 4.3% of patients (Lipsky et al., 1999).

18. Human-murine monoclonal antibodies

Infliximab is used to treat refractory Crohn's disease; in one patient suffering from lupus erythematous, insomnia was reported (Drosou et al., 2003).

19. Lipopeptide antibiotics

Daptomycin, a drug with bactericidal effects against Gram-positive bacteria has been reported to produce moderate neuropsychiatric effects such as headaches and insomnia (Gonzalez-Ruiz et al., 2011; FDA, 2003).

20. Metals

Antimony and arsenic: In observational studies, both antimony and arsenic caused insomnia in patients (Newlove et al., 2011; Takahashi, 2010). Insomnia was reported in 37.5% of people who were victims of chronic arsenic poisoning through drinking water in Mongolia (Guo et al., 2007).

21. Neuroleptics

The long-acting depot risperidone has a half-life of 3-6 days. Its most common adverse events include insomnia which is reported in 22.6% of patients (Louza et al., 2011). Insomnia was reported also as one of the common adverse effects of paliperidone in addition to extrapyramidal effects when used in patients with schizophrenia (Shim et al., 2008; Turkoz et al., 2011; Sliwa et al., 2011).

22. Norephinephrine re-uptake inhibitor (NRI)

Reboxetine-treated patients were more likely to experience constipation, difficulty urinating, and insomnia (Papakostas et al., 2008).

23. Opioid receptor agonists

Nalmefene, a drug used in order to promote abstinence in alcoholics, has been shown to induce insomnia in patients who received 20 micrograms per day (Anton et al., 2004).

24. Opioid analgesics

Insomnia has been reported as adverse event with dextromethorphan (Paul et al., 2004; Avis and Profile, 2005).

25. Selective serotonin reuptake inhibitor (SRRI)

Escitalopram, a selective serotonin reuptake inhibitor (SSRI) used in the treatment of major depressive disorder (MDD) and generalized anxiety disorder (GAD), has been reported to produce insomnia and decreased libido when used at 10 mg/day (Huska et al., 2007). In a large sample of 811 adult participants with depression in a part-randomised multicentre open-label study comparing escitalopram and nortriptyline, insomnia was reported in 36% of patients on escitalopram (Uher et al., 2009).

26. Smoking deterrent

In a review involving 120 studies (Mills et al., 2010), an increased risk of insomnia was associated with nicotine patch (OR 1.42, 95% CI, 1.21-1.66, $P < 0.001$)

27. Steroids

Insomnia has been reported in 27% of 103 patients treated for 8 days with more than 20mg/day of prednisone (Silverman et al., 1985; Aronson, 2010).

In an investigation of glucocorticoid-induced side effects in 68 Japanese patients treated for autoimmune diseases with prednisolone, insomnia occurred in 50% of them. It lasted on average 6 days, ranging from 1 to 88 days (Nakajima et al., 2009).

In case series of children with such discrete conditions as asthma and nephrotic syndrome, up to 50% of those receiving oral glucocorticoids have had adverse behavioural and affective effects including elevated levels of depression and anxiety, as well as increases in insomnia (Estrada de la Riva, 1958; Bender et al., 1988; Hall et al., 2003).

5. Strategies to manage drug-induced insomnia

Given the mechanisms of action described above, prescribers and dispensers of drugs should alert and inform the patients of the possibility that the drug they will be taking may lead to insomnia. For drugs that cause insomnia when withdrawn, the most common strategy has been to avoid abrupt withdrawal by tapering the dosing of the drug over several days (Lader et al., 2009).

For drugs that cause insomnia when being used, there are three strategies, namely, modification of dosage, discontinuation of drug, and switching to a different drug. When switching to a different drug, it is important to ensure that the insomnia as an adverse effect is not a "class-related effect" as shown above with regard to fluoroquinolones or cox-2 inhibitors. If so, a drug of a different class must be chosen or a drug that favourably enhances sleep should be considered as in case of salmeterol, a beta-adrenergic stimulator, that has been shown to improve quality of sleep. This medicine is recommended in asthmatics experiencing sleep disturbances (Lee et al., 2011; Nathan et al., 2006).

When insomnia occurs at a certain dosage level as in the case of prednisone, dosage reduction should be considered. This strategy is most relevant for the elderly. Generally, lower doses should be used in the elderly, although dose requirements may vary from person to person. Typically, starting doses for the elderly should be about one third to one half of the usual adult doses when a drug has a low therapeutic index or when another condition may be exacerbated by the drug (Kamal and Gammack, 2006).

With regard to preventing the occurrence of drug-induced insomnia, prescribers must be familiar with the drug and its potential adverse reactions. Drugs and initial dosage must be carefully selected for susceptible individuals such the elderly, those on cancer therapy, and children. Drugs which suppress slow-wave sleep (SWS) commonly leave the patient unrested; this might be counteracted by a sleeping medication that increases SWS, such as zopiclone. Clomipramine, a tricyclic antidepressant, may be used to suppress REM related nightmares. Both pharmacological and non-pharmacological treatment modalities should be explored in the management of drug-induce insomnia (Ellis et al., 2011; Foral et al., 2011).

6. Concluding remarks

Drug-induced insomnia is prevalent. It has been reported to occur to up to 50% of patients on specific drugs. While patients must be advised accordingly, precautions must be taken to avoid inducing insomnia through abrupt withdrawal of drugs, inappropriate dosing and irrational drug prescribing.

7. Acknowledgement

Thanks to Miss Mabjala R. Letsoalo who assisted with literature search.

8. References

Almay BG, von Knorring L, Wetterberg L. Melatonin in serum and urine in patients with idiopathic pain syndromes. Psychiatry Res 1987;22(3):179–191.

APA. Diagnostic and statistical manual of mental disorders, fourth ed. Washington, DC: American Psychiatric Association, 1994.

Ancoli-Israel S, Roth T. Characteristics of insomnia in the United States: results of 1991 National Sleep Foundation Survey. I. Sleep 1999;22(2):S347–S353.

Anton R, Pettinati H, Zweben A, Kranzler H et al. A multi-site dose ranging study of Nalmefene in the treatment of alcohol dependence. J Clin Psychopharmacol 2004;24:421-3

Aronson JK (Editor). Side effects of drugs. Annual 30. Elsevier, 2010

Avis R and Profile D. Dextromethorphan/quinidine AVP 923. Drugs R&D 2005;6(3):174-7.

Balter MB, Uhlenhuth EH. Prescribing and use of benzodiazepines: an epidemiologic perspective. J Psychoactive Drugs 1992; 24:63–64.

Baldwin CM, Kapur V, Holberg CJ. Rosen C, Nieto FJ. Associations between gender and measures of daytime somnolence in the Sleep Heart Health Study. Sleep 2004;27:305-11.

Benington JH, et al. A1 adenosine receptor stimulation mimics changes in non-REM sleep EEG slow-wave activity. Sleep Res 1993;22:4.

Ben-Menachem E, Edrich P, Van Vleymen B, Sander JW, Schmidt B. Evidence for sustained efficacy of levetiracetam as add-on epilepsy therapy. Epilepsy Res. 2003 Feb;53(1-2):57-64.

Ben-Menachem E, Gilland E. Efficacy and tolerability of levetiracetam during 1-year follow-up in patients with refractory epilepsy. Seizure 2003;12:31–5.

Bonnet MH, Arand DL. Impact of naps and caffeine on ex-tended nocturnal performance. Physiol Behav 1994;56(1): 103–109.

Baskett JJ, Wood PC, Broad JB, Duncan JR, English J, Arendt J. Melatonin in older people with age-related sleep maintenance problems: a comparison with age matched normal sleepers. Sleep 2001;24(4):418–424.

Bender BG, Lerner JA, Kollasch E. Mood and memory changes in asthmatic children receiving corticosteroids. J Am Acad Child Adolesc Psychiatry.1988;27:720-725.

Brugger P, Marktl W, Herold M. Impaired nocturnal secretion of melatonin in coronary heart disease. Lancet Jun;1995; 345(8962):1408.

Breslau N, Roth T, Rosenthal L, et al. Sleep disorders and psychiatric disorders: a longitudinal epidemiologic study of young adults. Biol Psychiatry 1996;39(6):411–4118.

Berkowitz R, Connelll J, Dietz A, Greenstein S et al. The effectiveness of the non-sedating antihistamine loratadine plus pseudoephedrine in common cold. Ann Allergy 1989;63(4):336-9.

Cajochen C, Krauchi K, Wirz-Justice A: Role of melatonin in the regulation of human circadian rhythms and sleep. J Neuroendocrinol 2003, 15(4):432-437.

Carvajal A, Arias LM, and Jimeno N. Antipsychotic drug. In Aronson JK (Editor): Side effects of drugs. Annual 29. Elsevier, 2007.

Chowdhury PP, Balluz L, Strine TW. Health-related quality of life among minority populations in the United States, BRFSS 2001-2002. Ethn Dis 2008;18:483-7.

Cohen PA, Benner C, McCormick D. Use of a Pharmaceutically Adulterated Dietary Supplement, Pai You Guo, Among Brazilian-Born Women in the United States. J Gen Intern Med. 2011 Aug 16. [Epub ahead of print]

Danel C, moh R, Anzian A, Abo Y et al. Tolerance and acceptability of an efavirenz-based regiment in 740 adult patients in West Africa. J Acquir Immune Defic Syndr 2006;42(1):29-35.

Dubocovitch M. Melatonin receptors: are there multiple subtypes? Trends Pharmacol Sci 1995;16:50–56.

Ellis JG, Gehrman P, Espie CA, Riemann D, Perlis ML. Acute insomnia: Current conceptualizations and future directions. Sleep Med Rev. 2011 May 17. [Epub ahead of print]

Espiritu j. Aging-related sleep changes. Clin Geriatr Med 2008 Feb;24(1):1-14.

Estrada de la Riva G. Psychic and somatic changes observed in allergic children after prolonged steroid therapy. South Med J. 1958;51:865-868.

Fekih L, Boussoffara L, Fenniche S, Megdiche M et al. Neuropsychiatric side effects of antituberculosis agents. Rev Med Liege 2011 Feb;66(2):82-5.

Fiorina P, Lattuada G, Silvestrini C, Ponari O, Dall'Aglio P. Disruption of nocturnal melatonin rhythm and immunological involvement in ischaemic stroke patients. Scand J Immunol Aug;1999;50(2):228–231.

Fick DM, Cooper JW, Wade WE, et al. Updating the Beers criteria for potentially inappropriate medication use in older adults: results of a US consensus panel of experts. Arch Intern Med 2003;163:2716-24.

Foral P, Dewan N, Malesker M. Insomnia: a therapeutic review for pharmacists. Consult Pharm. 2011 May;26(5):332-41.

Garfinkel D, Laudon M, Nof D, Zisapel N. Improvement of sleep quality in elderly people by controlled-release melatonin. Lancet Aug 26;1995 346(8974):541–544.

Garbutt JC, Kanzler HR, O'Malley S, Pettinati H et al. Efficacy and tolerability of long-acting injectable naltrexone for alcohol dependence. JAMA 2005;293(13):1617-25

Garcia-Escriva A, Lopez-Hernadez N et al. Lamotrigine in refractory epilepsy. Neurology 2004;63(2):373-5.

Gallant J, De Jesus E, Gazard B , Campo R et al. Tenofovir, emcitracitabine, and efavirenz versus zidovudine, lamivudine and efavirenz for HIV. N Engl J Med 2006;354(3):252-60.

Giannokodimos S, Georgiadis K, Tsounis S, Kimiskidis V et al. Add-on topiramate in the treatment of refractory partial-onset epilepsy: clinical experience of outpatient epilepsy clinics from 11 general hospitals. Seizure 2005;14:396-402.

Gorfine T, Assaf Y, Goshen-Gottstein Y, Yeshurun Y, Zisapel N: Sleep anticipating effects of melatonin in the human brain. Neuroimage 2006, 31(1):410-418.

Griffiths RR, Weerts EM. Benzodiazepine self-administration in humans and laboratory animals—implications for problems of long-term use and abuse. Psychopharmacology 1997;134:1-37.

Hajak G, Clarenbach P, Fischer W, et al. Rebound insomnia after hypnotic withdrawal in insomniac outpatients. Eur Arch Psychiatry Clin Neurosci 1998;248:148–156.

Hajak G, Rodenbeck A, Staedt J, Bandelow B, Huether G, Ruther E. Nocturnal plasma melatonin levels in patients suffering from chronic primary insomnia. J Pineal Res Oct;1995 19(3):116–122.

Hall AS, Thorley G, Houtman PN. The effects of corticosteroids on behavior in children with nephrotic syndrome. Pediatr Nephrol. 2003 Dec;18:1220-1223. Epub 2003 Oct 24.

Humbert W, Pevet P. Calcium content and concretions of pineal glands of young and old rats. A scanning and X-ray microanalytical study. Cell Tissue Res Mar;1991 263(3):593–596.

Hudson JI, David G Perahia, Inmaculada Gilaberte, Fujun Wang, John G Watkin and Michael J Detke. Duloxetine in the treatment of major depressive disorder: an open-label study. BMC Psychiatry 2007, 7:43. This article is available from: http://www.biomedcentral.com/1471-244X/7/43

Irwin M, Fortner M, Clarl C, et al. Reduction of natural killer cell activity in primary insomnia and in major depression. Sleep Res 1995;24:256.

Kales J, Kales A, Bixler EO, et al. Biopsychobehavioral correlates of insomnia. V: Clinical characteristics and behavioral correlates. Am J Psychiatry 1984;141(11):1371–1376.

Kamal and Gammack. Insomnia in the elderly: cause, approach and treatment. Am J Med 2006 Jun;19(6):463-9.

Kissel J, McDermott M, Mendell J, King W, Pandya S, Griggs R et al. Randomized, double-blind, placebo- controlled trial of albuterol in facioscapulohumeral dystrophy. Neurology 2001 Oct;57(8):1434-40.

Katz DA, McHorney CA. The relationship between insomnia and health-related quality of life in patients with chronic illness. J Fam Prac 2002;51:229-35.

Krystal AD. Treating the health, quality of life, and functional impairments in insomnia. J Clin Sleep Med 2007;3:63-72.

Kutner NG, Bliwise DL, Zhang R. Linking race and well-being within a biopsychosocial framework: Variation in subjective sleep quality in two racially diverse older adult samples. J Health Soc Behav 2004;45:99-113.

Kripke DF, Elliot JA, Youngstedt SD, Smith JS. Melatonin: marvel or marker? Ann Med 1998;30(1):81–87.

Jean-Louis G, Kripke DF, Ancoli-Israel S. Sleep and quality of well-being. Sleep 2000;23:1-7.

Lader M, Tylee A, Donoghue. Withdrawing benzodiazepines in primary care. CNS Drugs 2009;23(1):19-24.

Lancel M. Role of GABA-A receptors in the regulation of sleep: initial sleep responses to peripherally administered modulators and agonists. Sleep 1999;22:33–44.

Lee YS, Lin HC, Huang CD, Lee KY, Liu CY, Yu CT, Wang CH, Kuo HP.Efficacy and Tolerability of Salmeterol/Fluticasone Propionate versus Fluticasone Propionate in Asthma Patients: A Randomized, Double-blind Study. Chang Gung Med J. 2011 Jul-Aug;34(4):382-94.

Lieberman HR. Caffeine. In: Smith AP, Jones DM, eds. Hand-book of human performance,vol 2. Health and performance. San Diego: Academic Press, 1992:49–72.

Lipsky BA, Dorr MB, Magner DJ, Talbot GH. Safety profile of sparfloxacin, a new fluoroquinolone antibiotic. Clin Ther. 1999 Jan;21(1):148-59.

Lorist MM, et al. Influence of caffeine on information processing stages in well rested and fatigued subjects. Psychopharmacology 1994;113(3–4):411–421.

Lushington K, Dawson D, Kennaway DJ, Lack L. The relationship between 6-sulphatoxymelatonin and poly-somnographic sleep in good sleeping controls and wake maintenance insomniacs, aged 55–80 years. J Sleep Res Mar;1999 8(1):57–64.

Liu C, Weaver DR, Jin X, et al. Molecular dissection of two distinct actions of melatonin on the suprachiasmatic circadian clock. Neuron Jul;1997 19(1):91–102.

Marta Novak and Colin M Shapiro Drug-Induced Sleep Disturbances: Focus on Nonpsychotropic Medications. Drug Safety 1997; 16(2): 133-149.

McIntyre RS, Cohen M, Zhao J, Alphs L, Macek TA, Panagides J. Asenapine for long-term treatment of bipolar disorder: a double-blind 40-week extension study. J Affect Disord. 2010;126:358–365.

Merlotti L, Roehrs T, Zorick F, et al. Rebound insomnia: duration of use and individual differences. J Clin Psychopharmacol 1991;11:368–373.

Mendelson WB, Cain M, Cook JM, et al. Abenzodiazepine receptor antagonist decreases sleep and reverses the hypnotic actions of flurazepam. Science 1983;219:414–416.

Mendelson WB. Melatonin microinjection into the medial preoptic area increases sleep in the rat. Life Sci Sep 13;2002 71(17):2067–2070.

Mills EJ, Ping Wu, Ian Lockhart, Kumanan Wilson, Jon O Ebbert. Adverse events associated with nicotine replacement therapy (NRT) for smoking cessation. A systematic review and meta-analysis of one hundred and twenty studies involving 177,390 individuals. Tobacco Induced Diseases 2010, 8:8.

Mula M, Trimble M, and Sander W. Psychiatric adverse events in patients with epilepsy and learning disabilities taking levetiracetam. Seizure 2004;13(1):55-7.

Murphy PJ, Myers BL, Badia P. Nonsteroidal anti-inflammatory drugs alter body temperature and suppress melatonin in humans. Physiol Behav 1996;59(1):133–139.

Nakajima A, Doki K, Homma M, Sagae T, Saito R, Ito S, et al. Investigation of Glucocorticoid-induced Side Effects in Patients with Autoimmune Diseases. YAKUGAKU ZASSHI 2009; 129: 445-450.

Nathan P, O'Neill B, Napolitano A, Bullmore E. Neuropsychiatric effects of centrally-acting of antiobesity drugs. CNS Neurosci Ther 2010 Jul;

Nathan RA, Rooklin A, Schoaf L, Scott C, Ellsworth A, House K, Dorinsky P. Efficacy and tolerability of fluticasone propionate/salmeterol administered twice daily via hydrofluoroalkane 134a metered-dose inhaler in adolescent and adult patients with persistent asthma: a randomized, double-blind, placebo-controlled, 12-week study. Clin Ther. 2006 Jan;28(1):73-85.

Olsen RW, Tobin AJ. Molecular biology of the GABA-A receptor. FASEB J 1990;4:1469–1480

Papakostas GI, Nelson JC, Kasper S, Möller HJ. A meta-analysis of clinical trials comparing reboxetine, a norepinephrine reuptake inhibitor, with selective serotonin reuptake inhibitors for the treatment of major depressive disorder. Eur Neuropsychopharmacol. 2008Feb;18(2):122-7.

Paquette A, Gou P, Tannenbaum C. Systematic review and meta-analysis: do clinical trials testing antimuscarinic agents for overactive bladder adequately measure central nervous system adverse events? J Am Geriatr Soc. 2011 Jul;59(7):1332-9. doi: 10.1111/j.1532-5415.2011.03473.x. Epub 2011 Jun 30.

Qiu L, Feng HY, Huang X, Mo R, Ou CY, Luo CM, Li Y, Liu WB. [Study of incidence and correlation factors of depression, anxiety and insomnia in patients with myasthenia gravis]. Zhonghua Yi Xue Za Zhi. 2010 Dec;90(45):3176-9.

Redline S, Tishler PV, Hans MG, Tosteson TD, Strohl KP, Spry K. Racial differences in sleep-disordered breathing in African-Americans and Caucasians. Am J Resp Crit Care Med 1997;155:186-92.

Riemann D, Klein T, Rodenbeck A, et al. Nocturnal cortisol and melatonin secretion in primary insomnia. Psychiatry Res Dec 15;2002 113(1–2):17–27.

Richardson G, Tate B. Hormonal and pharmacological manipulation of the circadian clock: recent developments and future strategies. Sleep 2000;23 (Suppl 3):S77–85.

Rosenthal L, et al. Alerting effects of caffeine after normal and restricted sleep. Neuropsychopharmacology 1991;4(2):103–108.

Roehrs T, Zorick F, Roth T. Transient and short-term insomnias. In: Kryger M, Roth T, Dement WC, eds. Principles and Practice of Sleep Medicine. 3rd edition Philadelphia, PA: W.B. Saunders and Company; 2000:624–632.

Roehrs TA, Zorick FJ, Wittig RM, et al. Dose determinants of rebound insomnia. Br J Clin Pharmacol 1986;22:143–147.

Roth T, Ancoli-Israel S. Daytime consequences and correlates of insomnia in the United States: results of the 1991 National Sleep Foundation Survey II. Sleep 1999;22(2):S354–S358.

Roth T, Roehrs T. Insomnia: epidemiology, characteristics, and consequences. Clin Cornerstone. 2003;5:5–15.

Sack RL, Brandes RW, Kendall AR, Lewy AJ. Entrainment of free-running circadian rhythms by melatonin in blind people. N Engl J Med 2000;343(15):1070–1077.

Saddichha. Diagnosis and treatment of chronic insomnia. Ann Indian Acad Neurol 2010 Apr;13(2):94-102.

Salmon, S. E. and Sartorelli, A. C. Cancer Chemotherapy, in Basic and Clinical Pharmacology, (Katzung, B. G., ed) Appleton-Lange, 1998, p. 881-911.

Schwartz S, McDowell Anderson W, et al. Insomnia and heart disease: a review of epidemiologic studies. J Psychosom Res 1999; 47(4):313–333.

Sharma M, Palacios-Bois J, Schwartz G, et al. Circadian rhythms of melatonin and cortisol in aging. Biol Psychiatry 1989;25(3):305–319.

Sharpley AL, Cowen PJ. Effect of pharmacologic treatments on the sleep of depressed patients. Biol Psychiatry 1995;37:85–98.

Shochat T, Luboshitzky R, Lavie P: Nocturnal melatonin onset is phase locked to the primary sleep gate. Am J Physiol 1997, 273(1 Pt 2):R364-370.

Supiyaphun P, Chocahipanichnon L, Kerekhanjanarong V, Saengpanich S. A comparative study of the side effects between pseudoephedrine in Loratatine plus pseudoephedrine sulphate Repetabs and loratadine plus pseudoephedrine in the treatment of allergic rhinitis in Thai patients. J Med Assoc Thai 2002 Jun;85(6):722-7

Surrall K, Smith JA, Bird H, Okala B, Othman H, Padwick DJ. Effect of ibuprofen and indomethacin on human plasma melatonin. J Pharm Pharmacol 1987;39(10):840–843.

Stepnowsky C, Johnson S, Dimsdale J, Ancoli-Israel S. Sleep apnea and health-related quality of life in African American elderly. Ann Behav Med 2000;22:116-20.

Tanabe N, Fujita T, Fujii Y, and Orii T Investigation of the Factors that Contribute to the Onset of Insomnia in Hypertensive Patients by Using a Post-marketing Surveillance Database. YAKUGAKU ZASSHI 2011;131(5):669-677

Touitou Y, Fevre M, Lagoguey M, et al. Age- and mental health-related circadian rhythms of plasma levels of melatonin, prolactin, luteinizing hormone and follicle-stimulating hormone in man. J Endocrinol 1981;91(3):467–475.

Uher R, Farmer A, Henigsberg N, Rietschel M, Mors O, Maier W, Kozel D, Hauser J, Souery D, Placentino A, Strohmaier J, et al. Adverse reactions to antidepressants. Br J Psychiatry. 2009 Sep;195(3):202-10.

Van Den Heuvel CJ, Reid KJ, Dawson D. Effect of atenolol on nocturnal sleep and temperature in young men: reversal by pharmacological doses of melatonin. Physiol Behav Jun;1997 61(6):795–802.

Walsh JK, et al. Effect of caffeine on physiologic sleep tendency and ability to sustain wakefulness at night. Psychopharmacology 1990;101:271–273.

Wyatt JK, Dijk DJ, Ritz-de Cecco A, Ronda JM, Czeisler CA: Sleep-facilitating effect of exogenous melatonin in healthy young men and women is circadian-phase dependent. Sleep 2006, 29(5):609-618.

Youngstedt SD, Kripke DF, Elliott JA, Klauber MR. Circadian abnormalities in older adults. J Pineal Res Oct;2001 31(3):264–272.

Zammit GK, Weiner J, Damato N, et al. Quality of life in people with insomnia. Sleep 1999; 1(2):S379–S385.

Zhou Y, Wang X, Zeng X, Liu S et al. Positive benefits of theophylline in randomize, double-blind, parallel-group, placebo-controlled study of low dose, slow release theophylline in the treatment of COPD for one year. Respirology 2006 Sep;11(5):603-10.

Zhou JN, Liu RY, Van Heerikhuize J, Hofman MA, Swaab DF. Alterations in the circadian rhythm of salivary melatonin begin during middle-age. J Pineal Res Jan;2003 34(1):11–16.

Part 2

Clinical Issues, Diagnosis and Management

3

Specific Quality of Life Measures for Sleep Disorders

Sermin Timur and Nevin Hotun Şahin
Inonu University/School of Health,
Istanbul University/ Nursing Faculty,
Turkey

1. Introduction

Sleep is one of the most important needs for a healthy life. It is therefore considered to be an important aspect of health, affecting well-being and quality of life (Karadağ & Ursavaş, 2007; Léger & Bayon, 2010). Sleep disorders have been long to be known as a disease symptom. Recently, there has been a rapid increase in the number of studies on sleep disorders, which has come to be considered a problem or a syndrome in its own right. Insomnia is one of the most common sleep disorders and an important public health issue with high prevalence (Karadağ & Ursavaş, 2007; Léger & Bayon, 2010). 30% of the general population and 9-10% of the US population are affected by sleep disorders (Laar, et al., 2010; Roth, 2007). Insomnia is defined as the subjective perception of one's dissatisfaction with the amount and/or quality of sleep. It may manifest as difficulty in initiating or maintaining sleep or too early awakening and inability to return to sleep (Roth, 2007; Smolensky, et al., 2011).

Sleep disorders might cause life-threatening accidents, severe loss in work productivity, and disruptions in psychosocial functioning. Epidemiological studies indicate that sleep-related crashes represent up to 20% of all traffic accidents in industrial societies (Roth, 2007; Smolensky, et al., 2011). The literature suggests that sleeping difficulty doubles the risk of a fatal work-related accident (Scott, et al., 2011). Chronic insomnia has a negative impact on psychological well-being and quality of life. Almost 40% of the adults suffering insomnia were diagnosed with at least one psychiatric disorder, most commonly depression (Botteman, 2009; Laar, et al., 2010; Léger & Bayon, 2010; Roth, 2007).

2. Quality of Life (QoL) and Health-Related Quality of Life (HRQoL)

The concept of "quality of life" has a long history in the fields of sociology and medicine. Aristoteles, one of the earliest philosophers, dealt with the nature of happiness and the necessities of a 'good life'. For Aristoteles and most of his successors, the ultimate end of human life is achieving the highest good, that is attaining the best condition that one's life permits. In this way, an individual who achieves this goal has a life of highest quality. In the field of medicine, improving the well-being of patients was part of physicians' education, besides treating and curing their problems, as early as the times of Hippocrates (Müezzinoğlu, 2005).

After the World Health Organization (WHO) defined health positively as "a state of complete physical, mental, and social well-being and not merely the absence of disease or infirmity" in 1946, the interest in the concept of "Quality of Life (QoL)" has drastically increased. It is very difficult to make a precise definition of "Quality of Life", as it is a multifactorial concept covering several domains. The definition of quality of life changes from society to society as well as from individual to individual in a given society. According to general opinion, the following domains should be covered by the concept of Quality of Life: functional competence, complaints about illnesses and treatment, competence in psychological and social functioning. The World Heath Organization Quality of Life (WHOQOL) group defines quality of life as: "an individual's perception of their position in life, in the context of the culture and values in which they live and in relation to their goals, expectations, standards, and concerns". This definition focuses on the way patients evaluate their quality of life from their own perspective (Kyle, et al., 2010; WHO,1990).

Health-related quality of life (HRQoL) is an integral subcomponent of quality of life. These concepts are thus closely related. Following the general consensus, health-related quality of life could be defined as "the patient's own evaluation of the impacts of illness and treatment on themselves" (Kyle, et al., 2010; Müezzinoğlu, 2005).

The WHO model explains how the incompetencies resulting from various illnesses affect quality of life (Figure 1). Impairment is defined as a loss or abnormality of psychological, physiological or anatomical structure and function. Disability is a restriction or lack of ability to perform an activity in the manner considered normal for a human being. Handicap is defined as a condition resulting from an impairment or a disability that limits the fulfillment of a role that is normal for an individual (given his or her age, gender, social and cultural background). The presence of these three factors eventually leads to disability and thus to a reduced quality of life by making them depend on others. Social well-being is a complex concept consisting of many aspects such as mutual family support, social activities and friendship, financial sufficiency, personal life (protection of privacy and preservation of abilities), individual success, sexual satisfaction and life philosophy (Müezzinoğlu, 2005).

Indeed, a PubMed search reveals that publications with the term 'Quality of Life' in the title or abstract has risen more than approximately three-fold in the last ten years (2001–2011: 114.736), relative to the previous decade (1991–2001:42.244) (Kyle, et al., 2010; Müezzinoğlu, 2005). This increase is mainly caused by the important developments realized in the field of medicine, as a result of which most diseases have become curable, life span has increased, and everybody is now in a position to live with chronic diseases for longer periods. Patients' level of knowledge about illnesses and level of participation in the decisions concerning treatment have also increased inasmuch as communication possibilities have multiplied, and internet has become more accessible. Increased interest in the idea of "sanctity of life" in the field of medicine has also boosted the interest in the concept of quality of life.

Today, indicators such as reducing patient complaints and increasing life span are no longer sufficient to evaluate medical treatment. New criteria that take patients' perspective into account should be incorporated into the evaluation process (Müezzinoğlu, 2005; Kyle, et al., 2010). Moreover, HRQoL has become an important variable when deciding upon which treatment method to follow, how to use resources, and what type of service to provide (Kyle, et al., 2010).

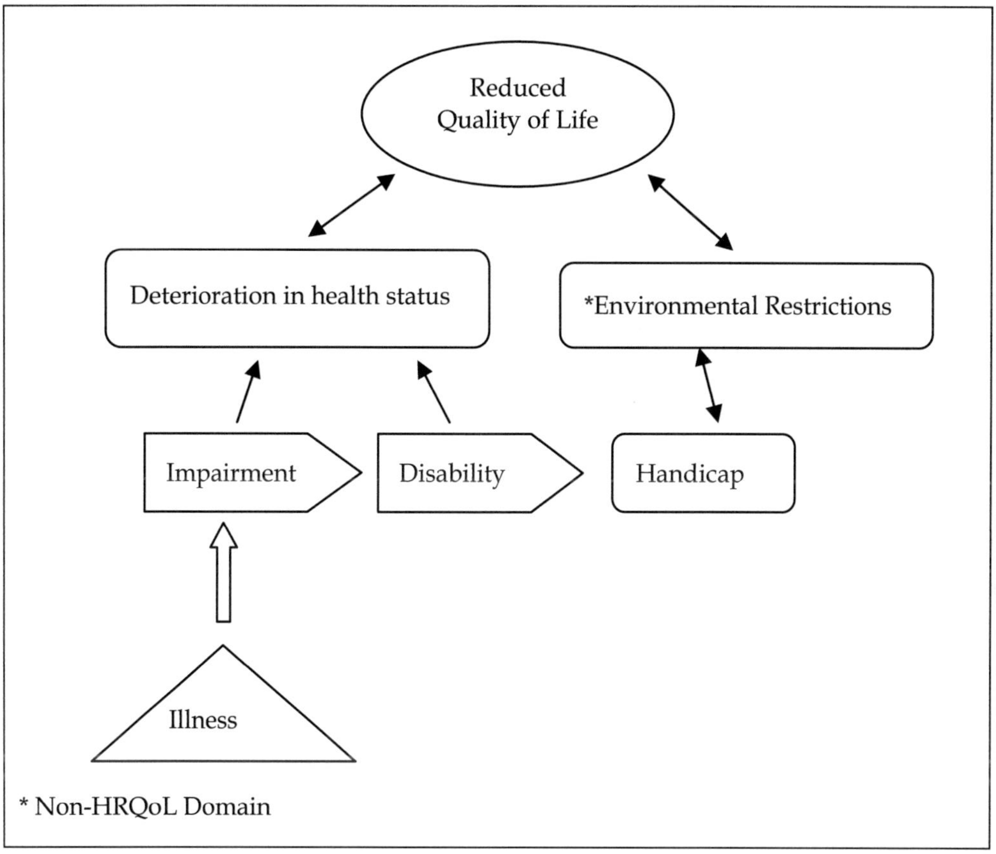

Fig. 1. The WHO model explains the interaction between the illness and the Qality of Life (WHO,1990)

Quality of life is essentially what individuals perceive as their overall sense of well-being based on functional ability, health, and satisfaction with the important dimensions of their lives. It is thus best determined in interaction with the individual. HRQoL measures could be divided into two main groups: generic and specific measures (Table 1) (Müezzinoğlu, 2005; Reimer & Flemons, 2003).

As generic scales comprise a broad spectrum of functional losses and general illnesses concerning HRQoL, they are applicable to all segments of society for all illnesses and are used in various medical practices. Generic scales are also divided into two sub-groups: "Health Profiles" and "Utility Measurement". Health profiles consist of a single scale and analyzes various aspects of health. It can compare different medical interventions. Possible disadvantage of these scales are unresponsiveness to small changes. Among the frequently used examples of generic measures are SF-36, the World Health Organization Quality of Life Scale (WHOQOL), Nottingham Health Profile, Functional Limitations Profile (FLP), Sickness Impact Profile (Table 1) (Müezzinoğlu, 2005; Reimer & Flemons, 2003; Weaver, 2001).

A-General Scales	Domains
A-1.Health Profiles	
SF-36	Physical functioning, Mental health (Psychological distress, Psychological well being), Role functioning, Social functioning, Health perceptions, Pain, vitality.
WHOQOL -BREF	Physical functioning, Mental health, Social functioning, Environment
Nottingham Health Profile	Physical functioning, Mental health (Psychological distress), Social functioning, Pain, vitality,sleep
Sickness Impact Profile	Physical functioning, Mental health (Psychological distress), functioning, Social functioning, Mobility/travel, sleep, Cognitive functioning, Eating, Recreation/hobbies, Communication, Home management
Functional Limitations Profile (FLP)	Physical functioning, Mental health (Psychological distress), functioning, Social functioning, Mobility/travel, sleep, Cognitive functioning, Eating, Recreation/hobbies, Communication, Home management
A.2.Efficacy Measurements	
The self-administered form of the QWB (QWB-SA)	mobility, physical activity, and social activity
EuroQol Instrument / EQ5-D	mobility, self-care, usual activities, pain/discomfort, and anxiety/depression
Health Utility Index-HUI	vision, hearing, speech, ambulation, dexterity, emotion, cognition, pain, self-care, pain, and fertility
B-Specific Scales	
B.1. Spesific Quality Of Life Measures for Sleep Disorders	
Ferrans and Powers	Health, function, socioeconomic, psychological/spiritual, and family
Functional Outcomes of Sleep Questionnaire (FOSQ)	activity level, vigilance, intimacy and sexual relationships, general productivity, and social outcome
Sleep Apnoea Quality Of Life Index (SAQLI)	Daily functioning, social interactions, emotional func tioning, symptoms, and treatment-related symptoms, which is applicable following the initiation of treatment.
The OSA Patient-Oriented Severity Index (OS APOSI)	sleep problems, awake problems, medical problems, emotional and personal problems, and occupational problems associated with OSA

Table 1. Distribution of Quality of Life Scales across Domains

Having been developed in light of various theories in the field of health economics, utility measurement scales are used for cost utility analyses, and most importantly for calculating quality-adjusted life year (QALY). HRQoL is reduced to a single score between '0' and '1'. It is very difficult to identify the utility values, and these scales cannot determine different aspects of quality of life. Like health profiles, utility measurement profiles cannot identify small changes either. Among the most frequently used utility measurement scales are the self-administered form of the QWB (QWB-SA), the Europe Quality of Life Instrument (EuroQol Instrument / EQ5-D) and the health utility index (Health Utility Index-HUI) (Table 1) (Müezzinoğlu, 2005; Reimer & Flemons, 2003; Weaver, 2001).

Specific measures, however, are clinically sensitive and can identify small changes. On the other hand, being dependent on the group or intervention to which the measure would be applied is a disadvantage of specific measures. It cannot compare different situations. Measures could be specific to a particular population segment: children, seniors, adults. There is a specific measure for almost all diseases (epilepsy, diabetes, rheumatoid arthritis), conditions (pain), and functions (sexual function, emotional status, and sleep) (Table 1) (Müezzinoğlu, 2005; Reimer & Flemons, 2003; Weaver, 2001).

3. Specific Quality Of Life Measures for Sleep Disorders

Insomnia affects the daily lives of sufferers. Quality of Life is an effective instrument of measurement to calculate the impact of insomnia on daily functions. Sleep disorder specific measures of quality of life among insomniacs are quite few (Léger & Bayon, 2010; Reimer & Flemons, 2003). It is stated that there is a need for more sleep disorder specific quality of life measures. Among the well-known examples of such measures are the Ferrans and Powers Sleep Disorder Specific Quality of Life Index, the Functional Outcomes of Sleep Questionnaire (FOSQ), the Calgary Sleep Apnea Quality of Life Index (SAQLI), and the OSA Patient-Oriented Severity Index (OS-APOSI) (Léger & Bayon, 2010; Reimer & Flemons, 2003).

3.1 The Ferrans and Powers sleep disorder specific Quality of Life Index

Ferrans and Powers developed one of the first sleep disorder specific quality of life measures for use in narcolepsy. They adapted this specific measure from their own generic quality of life measure. The Ferrans and Powers index has four domains; health and function, socioeconomic, psychological/spiritual, and family. Each domain and the total score have a range of 0 to 30, calculated by averaging all the item scores. However, the sleep disorder specific quality of life measure has not been much adopted (Reimer & Flemons, 2003; Flemons & Reimer, 2002).

3.2 Functional Outcomes of Sleep Questionnaire (FOSQ)

The Functional Outcomes of Sleep Questionnaire (FOSQ) is a functional instrument of measurement to identify the impacts of intense sleep disorders on social, mental and physical functions required in daily activities (Reimer & Flemons, 2003). The questionnaire aims to identify whether an individual is having difficulties performing daily activities when they feel tired or sleepy. In this questionnaire, "sleepy" and "tired" indicates inability to keep one's eyes open, having a droopy head or feeling an urge to take a nap (Şengül et al., 2011; Reimer & Flemons, 2003). The questionnaire consists of 30 questions and 5 subscales, namely activity level, vigilance, intimacy/sexual relationships, general productivity, and social outcome (Reimer & Flemons, 2003). There are five possible answers for each question: no difficulty, a little, moderate, or extreme. Total score and subscale scores are calculated by summing up participants' answers. The intimacy/sexual relationships subscale is a unique feature of the FASQ. Despite having important consequences in the long run, this subscale is often confused with sleep disorder, and the significance of this life experience is often underestimated. The weakness of this subscale is that some participants are unwilling to respond to the questions or do not engage in sexual activities. One of the strengths of the subscale is that it excludes all factors except insomnia from analysis. Being used with SF-36, the FASQ is gaining popularity in the field. Successful testing of a Spanish version of the FASQ has been reported (Reimer & Flemons, 2003; Weaver, 2001).

3.3 Sleep Apnea Quality Of Life Index (SAQLI)

The Calgary Sleep Apnea Quality of Life Index (SAQLI) was developed as an evaluative instrument to measure within-subject change in response to a therapeutic intervention. The first 35 questions measure four domains: daily functioning, social interactions, emotional functioning, and symptoms (Flemons & Reimer, 2002; Reimer & Flemons, 2003).

The SAQLI use a 7-point Likert scale ranging from 1 (maximal impairment) to 7 (no impairment). Domain scores are averaged by dividing the total score by the number of questions answered, and the total score is averaged over the four domains so that all scores maintain a total range of 1 to 7. The SAQLI includes a fifth domain, to capture some of the adverse consequences of currently available therapies for sleep apnea. This fifth domain, comprising treatment-related symptoms, is used after a therapeutic intervention, and is subtracted from the other four domains in determining the total SAQLI score (Flemons & Reimer, 2002; Reimer & Flemons, 2003). Later, a shorter version of SAQLI form was developed, which could be filled in by the participants themselves. This shorter version of SAQLI was composed in light of the original SAQLI and the results of a clinical study (Reimer & Flemons, 2003; Weaver, 2001). Items were selected on the basis of their responsiveness, repeatability, readability, and representativeness of each of the first three domains. In order to make it easier for the participants to fill in the forms by themselves, "symptoms", which is the fourth domain, was replaced by the most commonly answered questions in the original SAQLI. Following the original SAQLI, a final question was added to the short SAQLI. Preliminary results show that the short SAQLI is as successful as the original SAQLI (Reimer & Flemons, 2003). In a study identifying the measurement characteristics of the Calgary Sleep Apnea Quality of Life Index (Measurement Properties of the Calgary Sleep Apnea Quality of Life Index), Flemons and Reimer (2002) evaluated quality of life using SAQLI, SF-36 and the Ferrans and Powers Index. They found that the SAQLI was closely related to other measures of quality of life and that it makes perfect measurements (Flemons & Reimer, 2002).

In a study comparing two health-related quality of life questionnaires among patients with sleep apnea, namely the Calgary Sleep Apnea Quality of Life Questionnaire (SAQLI) and the Functional Outcomes of Sleep Questionnaire (FOSQ), Kasibowska-Kuźnia et al. (2004) found that both measures had a Cronbach's alpha of 0.94 and verified their reliability. Even though both measures produced similar results, SAQLI was found to be more sensitive than the FOSQ. Their study also proves that the Polish version of the FOSQ is a useful measure for assessing HRQOL among patients with SAS (Kasibowska-Kuźniar, et al., 2004).

3.4 The Obstructive Sleep Apnea (OSA) Patient-Oriented Severity Index (OS APOSI)

The OSA Patient-Oriented Severity Index (OS-APOSI) is a 32-item HRQL measure that surveys the sleep problems, awake problems, medical problems, emotional and personal problems, and occupational problems associated with OSA. The OS-APOSI has established internal consistency, but analyses of concurrent validity and test-retest reliability have not been reported (Weaver, 2001).

4. Insomnia and Quality Of Life

Sleep quality and quality of life are naturally related. For patients, the impact of the symptoms of sleep disorder on their quality of life is an important input in their decision to go on with the existing treatment or look for a new one. For physicians, the impact of sleep disorder on patients and their partners is an important input when setting up a treatment program. For researchers, quality of life measures are often a primary outcome variable (Reimer & Flemons, 2003).

The findings reported here suggest at least some quality of life domains are almost always affected when patients experience a chronic sleep disturbance (Reimer 2003). In a study conducted by Şahbaz et al. (2008), it was found that patients who had Obstructive Sleep Apnea had a lower quality of life than people who did not (Şahbaz, et al., 2008). Sleep quality and quantity should be routinely assessed in primary care because of its association with quality of life, including symptoms of fatigue, energy levels, daytime sleepiness, mental and physical functioning, family relationships, and even bodily pain (Reimer & Flemons, 2003). In a study examining the impact of Nocturia on the sleep quality and quality of life among male patients, Kim et al. (2011) found that Nocturia had an immense negative effect on health-related quality of life and sleep quality (Kim, et al., 2011). In a study analyzing the relationship between quality of life and sleeping difficulties among patients with chronic obstructive pulmonary disease (COPD), Scharf et al. (2011) found that most patients with COPD suffered sleeping difficulties and that disease-specific quality of life and sleeping difficulty were related (Scharf, et al., 2011).

The general impact of sleep on the quality of life of a healthy individual is underestimated. The quality and quantity of sleep depend on various factors like level of energy. Level of energy could be associated with many types of diseases. At least some of the generic measures should thus be included in the studies evaluating the impact of a disease on one's life. The number of generic measures evaluating positive health is quite low. It is suggested that quality of life scales that include positive health be used on the healthy population under normal daily circumstances (Reimer & Flemons, 2003).

There are very few articles showing the impact of insomnia on quality of life. Most of the articles evaluate the impact of insomnia on quality of life among cancer patients. A considerable number of studies analyze the relationship between quality of life and sleep disorders among patients with diabetes, depression, Parkinson's disease, chronic kidney failure, and Human Immunodeficiency Virus (HIV). Indeed, quality of life should be systematically used to evaluate the pharmacological and non-pharmacological methods of insomnia treatment. In a report on sleep published by the World Health Consensus, it was suggested that more studies be conducted on insomnia and quality of life. SF-36 is one of the most frequently used scales to evaluate quality of life (Parish, 2009; Léger & Bayon, 2010).

5. Quality of Life in the management of insomnia

Insomnia affects daily lives of millions of people all over the world. In the medical literature, a strong relationship is identified between sleep duration, mortality and morbidity (Bixler,

2009; Crowley, 2011; Léger & Bayon, 2010). Sleep disorders are considered to have a great impact on economy. In the United States, direct and indirect costs associated with insomnia exceed $100 billion annually (Botteman, 2009). Moreover, the number of evidence showing the relationship between insomnia and other public health issues such as depression, accidents and anxiety is steadily increasing (Léger & Bayon, 2010; Roth, 2007; Crowley, 2011). Approximately 20% of all motor vehicle accidents are associated with driver sleepiness (independent of alcohol) (Scott, et al., 2011). Sleep apnea, restless leg syndrome, shift work sleep disorders, hypersomnia have also been proved to have an important impact from a socio-economic perspective (Léger & Bayon, 2010; Roth, 2007; Crowley, 2011). Patients' family and colleagues could also be negatively affected by insomnia. There are many studies in the medical literature showing that treating sleep disorders increase quality of life (Moyer, et al., 2001; Scott, et al., 2011). Protective measures should be taken in order to underscore the benefits of a good night's sleep and to ensure regular sleep among high-risk individuals. Public authorities should pay more attention to sleep hygiene and education (Bixler, 2009; Léger & Bayon, 2010). In a controlled clinical trial study evaluating the effectiveness of the sleep hygiene education provided to the workers of Information Technology Company, Kakinuma et al. (2010) found that the education program did not affect workers' night's sleep but decreased afternoon sleepiness at work (Kakinuma, et al., 2010).

Insomnia could be prevented by taking simple measures if the factors making one more sleepy or lose one's sleep are carefully considered. Exercise, relaxation techniques, taking a warm shower and behavioral therapy methods should be preferred to medication in the management of insomnia (Morgenthaler, et al., 2006; Akdemir & Birol, 2003; Öztürk, 2004). In a randomized controlled trial study conducted by Reid et al. (2010), it was found that aerobic physical activity accompanied by sleep hygiene education increased the quality of life and sleep quality among insomniac patients (Reid, et al., 2010).

In a pretest-posttest study on patients diagnosed with primary insomnia, Houdenhove et al. (2011) analyzed the impact of cognitive behavioral therapy for insomnia on quality of life using SF-36. It was found that cognitive behavioral therapy increased physical and mental HRQoL. However, absence of a control group was a weakness of this study (Houdenhove, et al., 2011). Şengül et al. (2011) analyzed the impact of exercise on the sleep structure and quality of life among patients with obstructive sleep apnea syndrome (OSA) using the FOSQ and SF-36. In their experimental study, exercise was found to improve the quality of life and sleep structure among patients with mild to moderate sleep apnea (Şengül, et al., 2011).

The first step in the management of insomnia is to check whether there is a notable mental or organic problem underlying insomnia. If so, the problem should get the appropriate medical treatment. Subsequently, the risk factors that could cause insomnia should be identified. Another important responsibility of health professionals is to educate others about sleep hygiene. Moreover, misknowledge and unhealthy practices among patients should be identified and corrected. General principles of sleep hygiene are as follows:

- Do not rush to medication solutions for insomnia,
- Get up in good time and perform activities of daily living as usual regardless of how late you went to bed, and avoid sleeping during day time,
- Avoid alcohol, coke, coffee, tea and cigarette after dinner,
- Do physical exercises a few hours before bedtime but avoid exhausting activities 1-2 hours before sleep,

- Avoid using bed room for activities other than sleeping such as studying, watching TV etc.,
- Avoid heavy meals for dinner,
- Do not force yourself to sleep when you are not sleepy but try to engage in relaxing activities that does not require too much effort instead. Refrain from stimulating TV shows or books (American Sleep Association, 2007; Morgenthaler, et al., 2006; Özgen, 2001; Öztürk, 2004; Timur & Şahin, 2010).

6. Conclusion

In conclusion, insomnia is an important health problem with high prevalence rates. It affects daily life negatively and could be a symptom or cause of various diseases. Evaluation of quality of life plays a big role in identifying the level of impact that insomnia has on an individual. Generic as well as disease-specific instruments of measurement are needed to assess quality of life. Sleep disorder specific quality of life measures are insufficient. Health professionals should aim to increase patients' quality of life as well as manage their sleep disorders. However, preventive measures should be considered before medication solutions. Sleep hygiene education is one of the most important preventive measures to increase sleep quality, and therefore quality of life.

7. References

Akdemir, N. & Birol, L. (2003). *Internal Medicine, and Nursing Care.* (1. edition), Vehbi Koç Vakfı, ISBN 975-7078-19-0, İstanbul.

American Sleep Association (2007). Sleep Hygiene Tips. Web: http://www.sleepassociation.org/index.php?p=sleephygienetips.

Bixler, E. (2009). Sleep and society: An epidemiological perspective. *Sleep Medicine.* Vol.10, pp.3-6.

Botteman, M. (2009). Health economics of insomnia therapy: Implications for policy. *Sleep Medicine.* Vol.10, pp.22–25.

Crowley, K. (2011). Sleep and Sleep Disorders in Older Adults. *Neuropsychol Rev.* Vol.21, pp.41–53.

Flemons, WW. & Reimer, MA. (2002). Measurement Properties of the Calgary Sleep Apnea Quality of Life Index. *Am J Respir Crit Care Med.* Vol.165, pp.159–164.

Houdenhove, LV. Buyse, B. Gabriëls, L. & Bergh, OV. (2011). Treating Primary Insomnia: Clinical Effectiveness and Predictors of Outcomes on Sleep, Daytime Function and Health-Related Quality of Life. *J Clin Psychol Med Settings.* DOI 10.1007/s10880-011-9250-7.

Kakinuma, M. Takahashi, M. Kato, N. Aratake, Y. Watanabe, M. Ishikawa, Y. Kojima, R. Shibaoka, M. & Tanaka, K. (2010). Effect of Brief Sleep Hygiene Education for Workers of an Information Technology Company. *Ind Health.* Vol.48, No.6, pp.758-65.

Karadağ, M. & Ursavaş, A. (2007). Dünyada ve Türkiye'de uyku çalışmaları. *Akciğer Arşivi.* Vol.8, pp.62-66.

Kasibowska-Kuźniar, K. Jankowska, R. Kuźniar, T. Brzecka, A. Piesiak, P. & Zwierzycki, J. (2004). Comparative evaluation of two health-related quality of life questionnaires in patients with sleep apnea. *Wiad Lek.* Vol.57, No.5-6, pp.229-32.

Kim, SO. Choi, HS. Kim, YJ. Kim, HS. Hwang, IS. Hwang, EC. Oh, KJ. Jung, SI. Kang, TW. Kwon, D. Park, K. & Ryu, SB. (2011). Impact of Nocturia on Health-Related Quality of Life and Medical Outcomes Study Sleep Score in Men. *Int Neurourol J.* Vol.15, pp.82-86.

Kyle, SD. Morgan, K. & Espie, CA. (2010). Insomnia and health-related quality of life. *Sleep Medicine Reviews.* Vol.14, pp.69–82.

Laar, MV. Verbeek, I. Pevernagie, D. Aldenkamp, A. & Overeem, S. (2010). The role of personality traits in insomnia. *Sleep Medicine Reviews*. Vol.14, pp.61–68.

Léger, D. & Bayon, V. (2010). Societal costs of insomnia. *Sleep Medicine Reviews*. Vol.14, pp.379–389.

Morgenthaler, T. Kramer, M. Alessi, C. Friedman, L. Boehlecke, B. Brown, T. Coleman, J. Kapur,V. Lee-Chiong, T. Owens, J. Pancer, J. & Swick, T. (2006). Practice parameters for the psychological and behavioral treatment of insomnia: an update. An american academy of sleep medicine report. *Sleep*. Vol.29, No.11, pp.1415-9.

Moyer, CA. Sonnad, SS. Garetz, SL. Helman, JI. & Chervin, RD. (2001). Quality of life in obstructive sleep apnea: a systematic review of the literature. *Sleep Med*. Vol,2, No.6, pp.477-91.

Müezzinoğlu, T. (2005). Quality of life. *Üroonkoloji Bülteni*. Vol.1, pp.25-29.

Özgen, F. (2001). Uyku ve uyku bozuklukları. *Psikiyatri Dünyası*. Vol.5, pp.41-48.

Öztürk, MO. (2004). *Sleep Disorders*. Ruh Sağlığı ve Bozuklukları. (10. edition), ISBN 975-93453-0-7, Nobel Tıp Kitabevleri, İstanbul, pp.64-65.

Parish, JM. (2009). Sleep-related problems in common medical conditions. *Chest*. Vol.135, No.2, pp.563-72.

Reid, KJ. Baron, KG. Lu, B. Naylor, E. Wolfe, L. & Zee, PC. (2010). Aerobic exercise improves self-reported sleep and quality of life in older adults with insomnia. *Sleep Med*. Vol.11, No.9, pp.934-40.

Reimer, MA. & Flemons, WW. (2003). Quality of life in sleep disorders, *Sleep Medicine Reviews*. Vol.7, No.4, pp. 335–349.

Roth, T. (2007). Insomnia: Definition, Prevalence, Etiology, and Consequences. *Journal of Clinical Sleep Medicine. Vol. 3, No. 5, pp.7-10.*

Scharf, SM. Maimon, N. Tuval, TS. Scharf, BJB. Reuveni, H. & Tarasiuk, A. (2011). Sleep quality predicts quality of life in chronic obstructive pulmonary disease. *Int J Chron Obstruct Pulmon Dis*. Vol.22, No.6, pp.1–12.

Scott, GW. Scott, HM. O'Keeffe, KM. & Gande, PH. (2011). Insomnia - treatment pathways, costs and quality of life. *Cost Effectiveness and Resource Allocation*. Vol.9, No.10, Doi:10.1186/1478-7547-9-10.

Sengül, YS. Ozalevli, S. Oztura, I. Itil, O. & Baklan, B. (2011). The effect of exercise on obstructive sleep apnea: a randomized and controlled trial. *Sleep Breath*. Vol.15, No.1, pp.49-56.

Smolensky, MH. Di Milia, L. Ohayon, MM. & Philip, P. (2011). Sleep disorders, medical conditions, and road accident risk. *Accident Analysis and Prevention*. Vol.43, pp. 533–548.

Şahbaz, S. Itil, O. Inönü, H. Öztura, İ. Yemez, B. Baklan, B. Etikan, I. & Seyfikli, Z. (2008). Quality of Life, Frequency of Anxiety and Depression in Obstructive Sleep Apnea Syndrome. *Tur Toraks Der*. Vol.9, pp.141-5.

Timur, S. & Şahin, NH. (2010). Menopause and Sleep. *Maltepe Üniversitesi Hemşirelik Bilim ve Sanatı Dergisi*, Vol.3, No.3, pp.61-66.

Weaver, TE. (2001). Outcome measurement in sleep medicine practice and research. Part 1: assessment of symptoms, subjective and objective daytime sleepiness, health-related quality of life and functional status. *Sleep Medicine Reviews*, Vol.5, No.2, pp. 103–128.

World Health Organization (1990). Internationale classification of impairments, disabilities and handicaps: A manual of classifications relating to the conseqences of disease. Geneva: WHO.

4

Fatigue

Per Hartvig Honoré
Department of Pharmacology and pharmacotherapy, Farma, University of Copenhagen, Denmark

1. Introduction

1.1 The characteristics of fatigue

Many severely ill patients are afflicted with severe symptoms from both the disease and from treatment. The symptoms encompass not only physical incapacity but they also have a psychological impact, which seriously may hamper the daily living of the patient as well as the social situation (Curt et al., 2000). In cancer patients, pain and emesis is still a burden to the patients (Jacobsen et al., 1999; Patrick et al.,) although new treatment algorithms have been introduced that alleviates these symptoms so that fatigue at present is the most common and worst experienced symptom, afflicting up to 90 % of patients with cancer (Irvine et al, 1994.; Beam, & Richardson. 1996; Irvine et al, 1994; Hartvig et al., 2006a; Hartvig et al., 2006b). Fatigue is a French word with no absolute correspondence to English or many other languages. This symptom is distinct from typical tiredness experienced by healthy individuals as a result of normal daily life which is relieved by rest. Fatigue is described by the patients as a tiredness that *"is worse than they have ever experience before"*, that makes them *"totally exhausted"* and *"unable to do even simple tasks"* (Curt et al., 2000).

Fatigue is a subjective multidimensional experience. It has various meanings in the scientific literature in which a common definition of fatigue is: "Fatigue is experienced as a subjective and internal feeling that appears not to be the same for everyone" (Ream & Richardson, 1996). According to the definition used by the National Comprehensive Cancer Network (NCCN) Fatigue Guidelines Committee, fatigue both refers to the physical and mental dimensions: "Fatigue is an unusual, persistent and subjective sense of tiredness related to e.g. cancer, or cancer treatment, that interferes with usual functioning" (Mock et al., 2000). Fatigue is associated with impairment of quality of life and thereby has a major impact on the patient, with significant consequences that may persist for a long period of time after completing treatment (Curt et al., 2000). Fatigue usually differs from excessive tiredness experienced by healthy individuals and is not relieved by rest or sleep.

Fatigue can be distinguished into mental and physical fatigue. The physical sensation of fatigue makes the patient unable to perform normal tasks due to the unusual feeling of tiredness. The mental fatigue could be experienced as emotional sensations e.g. decreased motivation, low mood and cognitive impairments and lack of concentration, respectively (Glaus et al., 1996; Ream & Richardson, 1997). The unusual character of cancer-related fatigue is described by a patient after therapy as: *"Now I feel just fine. That day I felt tired I did everything as I usually do, but every time I sat down, I only wanted to lie down and sleep"* (Adnan et al., 2010).

Fatigue can be acute or chronic. Acute fatigue is defined as intermittent, with rapid onset and only lasting for a short period of time (Wilson et al., 1994). Fatigue is perceived as chronic if it lasts for more than six months. Different studies have revealed that chronic fatigue may improve with time but that it mostly persists for many years (Wilson et al., 1994). This in turn has a major negative impact on the patients quality of life (Curt et al., 2000; Diaz et al., 2008). Several factors contribute to the experience of fatigue, and the influence and perception of each factor may vary from patient to patient, adding further complexity to the diagnosis. A lot of research has highlighted the correlation of physiological and psychological factors with the severity of fatigue (Hwang et al., 2003; Diaz et al., 2008). The mechanisms that cause fatigue in patients e.g. with cancer are not completely known but may be related to release of cytokines causing stress to the brain (Hartvig-Honoré., 2010).

1.2 Prevalence of fatigue as studied in cancer patients.

Fatigue seems to be a more frequent part of the symptom complex in certain types of cancer. Consistent among studies, lung cancer patients may experience the highest degree of fatigue (Richardson, 1995; Yennurajalingam et al., 2008). Patients with a diagnosis of prostate-, lymphoma- and gynecologic cancer stated that they experienced less fatigue before treatment for the cancer than during treatment (Hartvig et al., 2006a). For the gynecologic patients it was not expected that they were less tired during treatment than before, although they still experienced rather high degree of fatigue as a group. This result could be due to regression of their tumors. Women with breast cancer also reported fatigue before start of treatment (Jong et al., 2004). In compliance with this, other studies dealing with breast cancer patients undergoing adjuvant therapy have also found fatigue prevalent at baseline (Ancoli-Israel et al., 2006). There is large heterogeneity in fatigue in patients with gynecological cancers. It was noted that patients with ovarian cancer should be separated from patients with cervix cancer, since a study indicated that patients with ovarian cancer experienced a severe fatigue while patients with cervix cancer experienced less of fatigue (Piper, 1993). The perception of fatigue is also gender specific as it has been shown that women experienced higher degree of fatigue than men (Cella et al., 1998).

1.3 Cytotoxic drugs may aggravate fatigue

In an observational study on the evolution of fatigue during cytotoxic drug therapy, a rapid increase to the worst fatigue scores was most common for all patients on the second and third days after initiation of cytotoxic drug treatment. Close to hundred percent of the patients reported fatigue after the start of cytotoxic drug administration, a finding that was consistent across studies (Pater et al., 1997: Jacobsen et al., 1999). After an initial increase of fatigue for the first two days after administration start, it gradually declined until the next treatment (Hartvig et al., 2006a). A study investigating fatigue severity throughout three treatment cycles has shown that fatigue remained stable for 48 hours after each cycle (Andrykowski et al., 2005). The findings confirm that fatigue is a significant clinical problem during administration of adjuvant cytotoxic drugs for many cancer patients (Hartvig et al., 2006a; Adnan et al., 2010).

While there is strong evidence that fatigue is most common during treatment, studies have also found a substantial number of breast cancer patients suffering from persistent fatigue even after treatment completion. Jacobsen et al. (2007) suggest that fatigue is a major issue for breast cancer patients becoming chronic in up to six months after completion of treatment. Another study showed an increased fatigue in up to 26% patients as compared to base-line levels post-treatment (Ancoli-Israel et al., 2006). This evidence confirmed that chemotherapy as a risk for developing fatigue that may continue long time even after treatment completion.

2. Contributing risk factors in cancer patients.

2.1 Type of cancer and treatment

There is a profound difference in the prevalence and severity in fatigue among cancer diagnoses as said. (Richardsson, 1995; Cella et al., 1998 ; Hartvig et al., 2006a; Hartvig et al., 2006b). This is both due to the cancer itself but also due to the cytotoxic drug regiment and to radiotherapy (Ahlberg et al., 2003) Breast cancer is the most studied patient population with large variations in severity due presence of contributing risk factors. (Jacobsen et al., 1997; Bower et al.; 2000).

2.2 Cytotoxic drugs

Analysis of cytotoxic drug regimens in an unselected group of patients revealed that the highest mean fatigue scores were experienced by patients from the first cycle who received in falling order: gemcitabine, cyclophosphamide, fluorouracil in combination, epirubicin (FEC), docetaxel, carboplatin and fluorouracil (Hartvig et al., 2006a; Hartvig et al., 2006b; Adnan et al., 2010). So far not any clear cut relationship between different cytotoxic drug regiments and the degree of fatigue has been truly established (Yennurajalingam et al., 2008). One study with a small number of patients in different treatment groups showed greater fatigue scores for subjects receiving bolus and continuous chemotherapy drugs as in the 5-flourouracil or the epirubicin, cisplatin and 5-fluorouracil protocol than for subjects receiving a short-term infusion every 21 days (Richardson et al., 1998).

2.3 Risk increase as co-morbidities, age and co-concomitant medicine

2.3.1 Kidney function

There are few studies that relate co-morbidities in patients to fatigue. In a study on hematologic malignancies, Kim et al. (2008) found that patients suffering from a kidney disease were more likely to report fatigue.

Studies have previously suggested that fatigue may be caused by elevated inflammatory activity. Additionally, kidney and hepatic function impairment could also be caused by inflammatory autoimmune disorders, which suggest a correlation between fatigue and impairment of kidney or hepatic function impairment. Another study on patients with haematological malignancies found that fatigue did neither correlate with inflammatory activities, nor with renal or hepatic function (Dimeo et al., 2004).

2.3.2 Age

Fatigue is more often and more severe in younger patients. Elderly women reported also less fatigue than the younger women did and young age is considered a risk factor for fatigue (Cella et al., 1998).

2.4 Co-related symptoms

Fatigue seems to be a most prominent and aggravating symptom experienced by a large majority of patients. Investigations carried out with heterogeneous groups of cancer patients (Hartvig et al., 2006a; Hartvig et al., 2006b) showed that fatigue appear to be one of the most frequently reported side effects. Evidence suggests that cancer-related fatigue is often accompanied by other bothersome adverse effects (Pud et al., 2008; Yamagishi et al., 2009).

A large scale research study was recently done identifying symptom prevalence and intensity in cancer patients receiving adjuvant chemotherapy (Jacobsen et al,. 1999). It was found that fatigue was one of the predominant symptoms occurring in cancer. Other disturbing symptom was reported and was ranged in severity in the following order: fatigue > sleep disturbance > unrest > anxiety > diarrhea > depression > constipation and pain.

2.4.1 Insomnia

Insomnia, e.g. sleep disturbance with difficulties falling asleep, disrupted sleep and early awakenings are common together with other sleep difficulties may often co-exist with fatigue. Among these insomnia and hypersomnia which are found affecting 30 to 50%, respectively of patients (Berger et al., 1998; Liu et al., 2009). Insomnia was also significantly associated with fatigue (Hwang et al., 2003).

Insomnia and subsequent sleep disturbances can lead to fatigue, mood disturbances, and contribute to Immuno-suppression, which can have a profound impact on quality of life and perhaps affect the course of disease. Insomnia in cancer patients must be distinguished from cancer-related fatigue (O'Donnel, 2004). Although they are two distinct conditions, insomnia and fatigue are interrelated. Insomnia often leads to daytime fatigue that interferes with normal functioning. Conversely, daytime fatigue can lead to behaviors such as napping, which results in insomnia. Because insomnia in this patient population may be due to a variety of causes, treatment must be multimodal and include both pharmacologic and non-pharmacologic therapies as discussed below.

Factors involved in circadian activities and rest have been evaluated and it was found that women who were less physically active and had increased number of night awaking reported higher cancer-related fatigue during chemotherapy (Andrykowski et al., 2005). In other words, sleep disorders may often exacerbate fatigue. The causal interrelationship between fatigue and sleep disturbance makes it difficult to distinguish between them. This is due to the fact that both sleep disturbance and fatigue might be a result of each other. Both symptoms are found to be most prevalent and most common during treatment of e.g. cancer patients. (Jong et al.. 2004). Women with cancer are even likely to experience fatigue and sleep disturbance before receiving their cytotoxic drug treatment (Jong et al., 2004).

2.4.2 Depression

Symptoms resembling fatigue are part of the associated symptom complex in patients suffering from fatigue. Therefore an association between depression and fatigue is common (Jacobsen et al., 1999). Depression experienced by severely ill as well as cancer patients is not significantly different from depression related to other diseases and medical conditions. However there is great variation in the reported frequencies of depression. A study assessed depression during cytotoxic drug treatment, and it was found that patients suffer more from depression and other symptoms during treatment than before initiating treatment (Curt et al., 2000).

It is still unclear whether fatigue is a cause or a result of depression, as both symptoms are closely related (Jacobsen et al., 2007). A study examining the relation of cancer related symptoms and their co-occurrence on health related quality of life, found a 44% depression prevalence in out-patients with cancer (Hwang et al., 2003). An association between depression, anxiety and fatigue has been found (Jacobsen et al., 1999). This correlation was not maintained when fatigue increased.

2.4.3 Pain

Pain may also be a contributing factor to fatigue and affect adversely the quality of life. Cancer patients' experience of pain was found to be a major concern for most of them and had substantial impact on quality of life (Pud et al., 2008).

2.4.4 Emesis and nausea

Emesis and nausea are direct consequences of some treatment modalities. Just like pain, nausea and emesis are considered to be acute symptoms but manageable side effects that are most often palliated with antiemetic drugs. Studies have found that nausea and emesis contribute to fatigue severity (Diaz et al., 2008).

2.4.5 Anaemia

Anaemia may be a contributing factor to fatigue and so indirectly associated with an adverse impact on quality of life The correlation between anaemia and fatigue has been demonstrated by several studies (Romito et al., 2008). It is proposed that anaemia may be caused of either a consequence of the cancer disease or by the myelo-suppressive chemotherapy due to the elevation of cytokines IL-1, IL-6 and TNF which in turn suppress the production of red blood cells (Kurzrock, 2001). The severity of anaemia varies depending on the degree of the disease and the type of treatment that the cancer patient is undergoing.

2.4.6 Cachexia

Cachexia is among other symptoms also a factor associated with the development of fatigue (Kalman, 1997; Gutstein, 2001). The aetiology of cachexia is multi-factorial and the mechanisms attributable to the development are complex. Among these the accumulation of cytokine by-products occurs due to cellular damage, which interferes with the hypothalamic control of hunger. Loss of appetite caused by cachexia results in a decrease in muscle mass which then leads to weakness and weight loss. Cachexia decreases quality of life and the performance status.

2.4.7 Variation in fatigue and co-existing symptoms over time

A relation exists between rated fatigue and the rated severity of other symptoms following chemotherapy. A study has found that fatigue, insomnia, depression, pain and anxiety were all positively correlated with one another (Ahlberg et al., 2003). The close link between these symptoms suggests that common mechanisms could underlie their development. There is a high inter- and intra-individual variability in symptom severity including fatigue, a problem well-known from qualitative questionnaires.

3. Fatigue interference with quality of life

Development of fatigue is not only found to be the most frequently reported symptom but it has also a substantial impact on the patients' quality of life in cancer. Impairments in activity, work, concentration, socializing and mood are obvious. Fatigue interferences with the quality of life at the first week after chemotherapy administration followed by a decline the two next weeks (Curt et al., 2000, Diaz et al., 2008). It is noted that the ability to work, the activity level as well as concentration capability are equally affected during the first week.

The patients' perception of their exhaustion and how it interferes with their ability to concentrate and work was reported in a study interviewing patients receiving adjuvant treatment for breast cancer and statements are listed: *"I was probably more mentally worn out, which was why I have not worked so much. But I have still felt ok.* Another patient stated: *"There are some difficult concepts to work with. My situation offers concentrations difficulties, but I have doubts whether it is influenced by the amount of medication"* (Adnan et al., 2010) .

These findings indicate that higher activity and mood as well as the ability to work, socialize and concentrate are increased when fatigue is rated low. This evidence demonstrates that fatigue has a profound impact on quality of life including physical and psychosocial aspects. It also points to the importance of managing fatigue and all other factors contributing to its occurrence. It is observed that a high prevalence of fatigue together with sleep disturbances, anxiety, diarrhoea, depression, constipation and pain, correlates with a decrease in quality of life. Jacobsen et al. (2007) suggested that fatigue is a major problem negatively impacting cancer patients' quality of life. However, it should not be ruled out that the other symptoms besides fatigue may also contribute to the impairment of cancer patients' quality of life.

4. Mechanisms of fatigue

The patho-physiology of fatigue is still not well understood although fatigue symptoms following severe disease particularly cancer and cytotoxic drug treatment have been well-known since long. The molecular mechanisms behind fatigue were although recently proposed by Hartvig-Honoré (2010). A comparison of the symptomatology in permanent and transient disturbances of brain neuromodulation enhances the basic knowledge on regulation factors, e. g. depressive behavioural changes after exhausting exercise or in fatigue. This consideration includes that the interaction between altered central neuromodulation and peripheral metabolic or hormonal dysfunctions is able to initiate the symptoms (Aistars et al., 1987). It is suggested that the central neuromodulation disturbance of stress-induced symptoms initiates the manifestation of the impairment (Hartvig-Honoré, 2010).

The symptoms of fatigue are sometimes divided in those with a peripheral origin and those due to a stress of the brain (Hann et al., 1998). Both types of symptoms might be present simultaneously. Symptoms from peripheral exhaustion may depend on neuromuscular malfunction or are related to deficiencies in peripheral neurotransmission. These symptoms are often related to immunologic mechanisms induced by the disease as well as its treatment and are accompanied by a release of cytokines (Swain, 2000.) The cytokines may in turn cause "stress" to the brain and change central neurotransmission.

4.1 Peripheral changes of importance for fatigue

One of the theories claims that cancer- and cytotoxic induced fatigue is due to accumulation of various metabolites such as lactate, hydronium ions and cell destruction end products (Piper et al., 1987). Lactate production is increased in cancer. Hydronium ions formed from lactate accumulation may impede muscle force and reduce the number of active actinomycine interactions (Piper et al., 1987).

4.2 Effects of cytokines

Although it has not been definitely proven it is suspected that cytokines such as interleukins, interferon and tumour necrosis factor, TNF- α play a significant role in fatigue, (Blackwell & Christman, 1996). Elevation of the pro-inflammatory cytokines interleukin-1β (1L-1β), IL-6 and tumour necrosis factor TNF-α concentrations is observed in both cancer and its treatment (Blackwell & Christman, 1996; Altar, 1999). Significant correlations with fatigue have been observed for increased interleukin-1 concentrations in men under irradiation therapy for prostate cancer and similarly interleukin elevations were observed in lung cancer patients treated with cytotoxic drugs (Tartaglia & Goeddel, 1992). Cytokines are a category of protein-signaling molecules that are used extensively in cellular communication. The elevation of these cytokines triggers the manifestation of several symptoms such as fever, anaemia, cachexia as well as fatigue (Anisman et al., 1992). These cytokines are produced by macrophages, monocytes and dendrite cells and are also known to be linked to an altered nervous system (Cella et al., 1998; Bower et al., 2007). IL-6 has mainly been considered a pro-inflammatory protein, but there are several lines of evidence that it has anti-inflammatory actions as well (Chao et al., 1991). Of the anti-inflammatory properties of IL-6 function is to modulate pro-inflammatory response, increase C-reactive protein as well to increase cortisol concentrations (Steensberg et al., 2006). TNF-α blockade may reduce fatigue.

It is not known to what extent a peripheral increased interleukin release may affect brain function, but increased penetration over the blood-brain barrier or vagus stimulation are plausible suggested mechanisms. In turn, this may lead to effects on microglia activation and synapse function.

4.3 Changes of central neurotransmission

Fatigue may cause "stress" and alterations of several neurotransmitter systems in the brain. The transmitter systems usually discussed are the serotonergic and noradrenergic ones. Both these systems are closely linked to the control of corticotrophin releasing hormone, CRH release and hence patients with fatigue have an increased CRH sensitivity. Low brain concentrations of serotonin, norepinephrine and dopamine, but also an activated hypothalamic-pituitary-adrenal axis (HPA-axis) is linked to elevated glucocorticoid concentrations (Geinitz et al., 2001). In this way fatigue resembles key elements in depression and related disorders.

Cytokines are released in severe disease and during treatment (Kurzrock 2001). Of these, IL-1β, IL-2 and IL-6 have been of particular interest. Interleukins activate the hypothalamus-pituitary axis which controls CRH release (Steensberg et al., 2006), and is closely linked to serotonergic and noradrenergic neurotransmission. A close link between serotonin (5-HT) and TNF-α has been established and TNF-α may change the serotonin metabolism by increasing the neuronal release of 5-HT. Increase of 5-HT transport is seen, which thereby may decrease the concentration of 5-HT in the synaptic space. This feed-back loop between 5-HT and TNF-α might be dysfunctional in the case of increased cytokine release due to treatment. An increase in the functioning of the HPA-axis leads in addition to increased concentrations of cortisol, which in turn is controlled by the interaction of 5-HT with the HPA-axis (Larish et al., 2001; Bower et al., 2002; Morrow et al., 2002). Cytotoxic drugs as well as irradiation therapy impair the cell proliferation and may destroy endogenous microglia cells as well as hippocampus neurons and create an inflammatory response and impaired maintenance and control of the synapses (Bilbo et al., 2009).

4.4 Brain stress and corticotropin hormone release

Central fatigue symptoms are related to alteration in neurotransmitter function in the central nervous system, and accompanied by psychic distress seen as e.g. anxiety and depression (Hann et al., 1998). There are several hypothesis involved to explain the brain stress in fatigue. Stress can be described as non-specific and affecting any demand, activity or emotion and may lead to a state of alarm involving the sympathetic nervous system. Over extended time periods this depletes body reserves and a restoration system is necessary for protection (Aistars, 1987). According to other hypotheses, a system located in the midbrain and medulla of the brain may mediate stimuli that give rise to stress response. Inhibition of the system results in fatigue due either to inhibition of cortical activity due lowered sensory input or as a result of chronic stimulation of the system. (Aistars, 1987).

Stress and depression may decrease cortical input as well, but there are individual factors of great importance to resist the manifestations of the response. CRH in the brain and the HPA axis regulate stress and control the release of adrenocorticosteroid hormone, ACTH,"stress related hormone". CRH containing nerve fibres are projected to the hypothalamus and other brain centres. Studies in rats with a failing CRH release show pronounced alterations in these projections. Long term changes as in chronic disease show a suppression of the ACTH/CRH response both in animal models and in patients (Hann et al., 1998). Deterioration of neurones in the central nervous system e.g . hippocampus has been shown possible to repair by action of neurotrophic factors such as Brain Derived Neurotrophic Factor, BDNF (Hong et al., 1995).

4.5 The role of Brain Derived Neurotrophic factor in stress and exercise

One treatment remedy both in depression and fatigue is simple exercise. Exercise in the form of voluntary running has been shown to increase the concentration of mRNA of the neuron repairing- and neuro-protective substance Brain Derived Neurotrophic Factor, in the hippocampus, cerebral cortex and other areas of the brain (Mamounas et al., 2000; Swain et al., 2000). In contrast, acute stress decreases BDNF mRNA in the hippocampus (Adlard et al., 2004). BDNF may have a protective role in acute stress. Following immobilization, circulating corticosteroid concentrations were elevated and showed a reduction of the BDNF protein (Adlard et al., 2004). Rats given voluntarily access to running prior to the stress demonstrated significantly increased hippocampus BDNF as well as corticosteroid concentrations that remained high (Adlard et al., 2004). In animals without exercise the BDNF concentrations decreased shortly after stress. Thus, corticosteroids modulated the stress-related changes of the BDNF protein (Adlard & Cotman, 2004).

Exercise may override the negative effects of stress with remaining high concentrations of both corticosteroids and BDNF. Voluntary physical activity may, according to clinical observations and the study on treatment of cancer and cytotoxic induced fatigue (Adamsen et al., 2006; Andersen et al., 2006; Midtgaard et al., 2009) represent a simple non-pharmacological tool for maintenance of the neutrophin, e.g. BDNF concentrations in the brain. This hypothesis needs clinical validation, however.

There is a link to effect of exercise to serotonin regulation in the brain. Simple exercise has been a remedy for both cancer- and cytotoxic related fatigue and may give an exercise-induced increase of free tryptophan in blood due to liberation from albumin, which is caused by adrenergic induced lipolysis of free fatty acids and results in higher free tryptophan uptake into the brain. Consecutively enhanced serotonin biosynthesis may though not per se initiate mood improvement or battle central fatigue. In this context the neurodegenerative effect of kyuneric acid a metabolite of tryptophan has been implied as a further contribution to brain alteration playing a role in fatigue. Centrally originated fatigue, mental deficiency and behavioural alterations with depressive mood are probably not primarily caused by metabolic and neuromuscular alterations. The primary trigger of these transient behavioural alterations might instead be initiated by a central exhausting stress, which elicits impairment of complex neuromodulation, also afflicting the interaction of central neurotransmitters or hypothalamic neuropeptides as well as releasing factors. In a consecutive correction of the variation, the implication of the serotonergic system on the central neuromodulation disturbance might improve or prevent the progressive course both in transient and in permanent mental disorders. Similar mechanisms of a central stress might be implicated in fatigue, and might be battled by simple exercise due to a peripheral exhaustion (Adamsen et al., 2006; Andersen et al., 2006; Midtgaard et al., 2009).

Both an underlying disease and treatment may cause fatigue and they are hard to separate since they coexist. Many factors may contribute to subjective fatigue (Redeker et al., 2000, Hartvig Honoré, 2010)), and the exact mechanisms are not completely known. The contribution of each factor may vary between patients and in individual patients over the courses of illness and treatment. The degree of fatigue might also differ between diseases and cancer types (Hartvig et al., 2006a; Hartvig et al., 2006b).

5. Physical activity and fatigue

Physical exercise is often an intervention proposed in order to reduce fatigue. This evidence is congruent with the majority of studies investigating the relation between fatigue and physical activity (Midtgaard et al., 2009). A correlation between the number of days during which the patients have been active per week and fatigue prevalence was shown. It is noticed when number of physically active days increases it correlates with decreasing intensity of worst fatigue. Thus, it is noticed that fatigue is a major hindrance to physical activity (Schwartz, 2000).

Several studies support the benefits of physical exercise to manage fatigue during and after treatment. Breast cancer patients exercising on a regular basis showed a decrease in fatigue (Schwartz, 2000; Andersen et al.,2006). The apportioned outcomes of physical exercise during chemotherapy treatment resulted in decreased fatigue and hence improved quality of life. Voluntary exercise in rats has recently shown the same effect on BDNF (Adlard et al., 2004).

One of the essentials of managing fatigue is to give patients adequate information about physical exercise. This was surveyed by Hartvig et al (2006b) showing a significant decrease in fatigue severity after education information as compared to patients not provided with adequate information regarding physical activity. Not sufficient information was considered to be a hampering aspect in fatigue management. (Adamsen et al., 2006). It is important to carefully consider which type of exercise that may be most beneficial. The kind of physical activity is usually not investigated in surveys. Moderate intensity and tailored physical activities for each patient reduces fatigue significantly in cancer patients undergoing treatment (Adamsen et al., 2006).

6. Treatment targets for fatigue related syndromes

Modulation of interleukin release and control of different neurotransmitter systems in the brain as well as promotion of BDNF synthesis and release are new options to challenge fatigue. There are thus several targets for treatment of fatigue syndromes apart from the non-pharmacologic simple exercise. Since fatigue is accompanied by several other distressing symptoms, the recommended best treatment for fatigue is to treat all underlying symptoms such as insomnia, pain, diarrhoea, constipation, anaemia etc (Kalman, 1997). In particular anaemic patients, supplementation with erythropoietin and similars has been successful, but the intervention is more to support an underlying symptom of the fatigue (Demetri et al., 1998; Kim et al., 2008, Glasby et., 1997), although hippocampus neuron stimulation may be included among the effects. A further remedy is corticosteroids but they can only be used for a limited time.

6.1 Pharmacologic interventions

Pharmacological treatment has so far had limited success, but new principles should be further developed. The serotonin system is a target and contributor to the neurobiology of stress (Nitta et al., 1994). There are implications that the stimulation of the serotonin 5-HT_{2A} receptor mediates the increase (Rosel et al., 2000; Rumajogee et al., 2002), but also the decrease of corticosteroids (Sapolsky et al., 1990). Elevated concentrations of glucocorticoids are known to play a notable role in the stress-induced damage of the brain (Shirayama et al., 2002). Corticoids and acute or long-term stress are shown to depress the expression of the serotonin transporter and BDNF (van Loon et al., 1981., Stockmeier; 2003). There are indications that the stress-derived decrease of BDNF is mediated by the serotonin 5-HT_{2A} receptor. The down regulation of BDNF may contribute to the atrophy of neurons in response to stress. Several antidepressant treatments increase the mRNA concentrations of BDNF (Watanabe et al., 2003).

6.1.1 Brain derived neurotrophic factor

Infusion of BDNF itself in the brain creates antidepressant-like effects, and increases the concentration of serotonin transporter, serotonin and its metabolites. BDNF may in fact attenuate corticoid-induced neural cell death by producing regenerative sprouting of injured serotonergic nerve terminals (Adlard et al., 2004). In order to understand the stress induced fatigue and the depressant state, it is essential to reveal the mechanisms of which BDNF and corticoids regulate serotonin and 5-HT_{2A} receptor concentrations which may form new interesting targets to combat fatigue. There is information on the regulation of BDNF expression by different antidepressants or serotonin receptor agonists and antagonists (Piper et al., 1987), but there is a substantial gap in the knowledge of the regulatory effects of BDNF on the receptor level. In conclusion, a working hypothesis is that BDNF regulates the expression of 5-HT_{2A} serotonin receptors, and that corticoids may act negatively upon this action (Piper et al., 1987).

6.1.2 Serotonergic drugs

Treatment of fatigue with other serotonin modulating drugs has been tried such as serotonin re-uptake inhibitors and other antidepressant drugs but the effect was not satisfactory. Fatigue symptoms have also been managed by treatment with 5-HT serotonin receptor agonists. It is obvious that more selective tools for interaction in specific processes in serotonin turn-over and binding should be further explored. Psycho-stimulants enhancing serotonin concentrations have a short but limited time effect and the risks of tolerance, dependence and other side effects can not be overlooked

6.1.3 Cytokines

Cytokine treatment causes fatigue. Intervention in the interleukin balance might be another target for treatment. It is obvious that IL-6 also has anti-inflammatory actions thereby causing a feed back effect (Steensberg et al., 2006). In fact the time course of IL-6 closely corresponds to the timing of fatigue after cytotoxic drug treatment (Tartaglia & Goeddel, 1992) and may therefore have a positive effect on fatigue.

6.1.4 Future perspectives for treatment

Recently the causes and consequences of fatigue have been more focused seemingly because it is a devastating state and most suffering in many diseases. The interest has been pointed both to peripheral and to central mechanisms to explain fatigue. It is likely that different mechanisms may interact and aggravate the problem, meaning that multimodal treatments must be tried. Normal sleep seems to be a mainstay as in other depressive and exhaustion disorders. Patients with fatigue often experience a disrupted sleep and an early awakening. So far exercise is the most promising algorithm which seems contradictory in a state with severe exhaustion and tiredness. The pedagogic message to the patient should be that by exercise they may get a muscle tiredness that may successfully combat the brain excitation due to the fatigue stress and may cause tiredness to the brain. Simultaneously, other signs that aggravate fatigue must be treated (Kalman, 1997). At present a curing pharmacological treatment for fatigue seems not possible.

7. Conclusions

Fatigue is a significant clinical problem during chemotherapy in cancer. As a confirmation to this, 100% of breast cancer patients have reported to experience fatigue immediately after the start of chemotherapy treatment. Cancer patients even report fatigue at baseline followed by a statistically significant increase in fatigue severity after treatment initiation. The chemotherapy induced fatigue is transient as the fatigue declines at the end of treatment cycle as the patients are slowly recovering.

Chemotherapy induced fatigue is found to be a more predominant symptom occurring as compared to others like sleep disturbance, being more prevalent than unrest > anxiety > diarrhea > depression > constipation and pain. A close time relation between the different symptoms and fatigue may be observed throughout the treatment. This evidence points to the complexity of managing fatigue due to its co-relation with other symptoms. Further risks for fatigue are young age, female gender and type, length and severity and type of tumor disease as well as type of chemotherapy drugs used and concomitant radiotherapy. Fatigue had a major impact on patient's quality of life on the daily basis comprising both physical and psychological aspects. All these findings confirm the multi-dimensional nature of fatigue and emphasize the importance of a multimodal treatment approach. Successful treatment algorithms are not many so far. Apart from careful management of all co-existing symptoms, only a moderate daily exercise has found some impact on the symptom with earlier vanish of fatigue but also less disturbing symptoms.

8. Acknowledgement

The author declares no conflicts of interest.

9. References

Adamsen, L., Quist, M., Midtgaard, J., Andersen, C., Moller, T., Knutsen, L., Tveteras, A. & Rorth, M. (2006) The effect of a multidimensional exercise intervention on physical capacity, well-being and quality of life in cancer patients undergoing chemotherapy. *Support. Care Cancer* 14, 116-127.

Adlard, P.A., & Cotman, C.W. (2004) Voluntary exercise protects agains stress induced decreases in brain derived neutrophic factor protein expression. *Neurosci.*, 124, 985-992.

Adnan, A., Hartvig Honore P., & Brix Tange U. (2010) Risk prevalence of cancer and cytotoxic induced fatigue. *Farmacja Onkolologiza*, (Oncol Pharmacy in Poland), 3, 16, 23-30.

Ahlberg, K., Ekman, T., Gaston-Johansson, F. & Mock. V. (2003) Assessment and management of cancer-related fatigue in adults. *The Lancet*, 362, 640-650.

Aistars, J. (1987) Fatigue in cancer patients: a conceptual approach to a clinical problem. *Oncol. Nurs. Forum*, 14, 6, 25-30.

Altar, C.A. (1999) Neutrophins and depression. *Trends Pharmacol. Sci*, 20, 59-61.

Ancoli-Israel, S., Liu, L., Marler, M.R., Parker, B. A., Jones, V., Sadler, G. R., Dimsdale, J., Cohen-Zion, M. & Fioren-tino, L. (2006) Fatigue, sleep, and circadian rhythms prior to chemotherapy for breast cancer. *Support. Cancer Care*, 14, 201-209.

Andersen, C., Adamsen, L., Moeller, T., Midtgaard, J., Quist, M., Tveteraas, A. et al. (2006) The effect of a multidimensional exercise program on symptoms and side-effects in cancer patients undergoing chemotherapy - the use of semi-structured diaries. *Eur. J. Oncol. Nurs.*, 10, 247-262.

Andrykowski, M. A., Schmidt, J. E., Salsman, J. M., Beacham, A. O. & Jacobsen, P. B. (2005) Use of a case definition approach to identify cancer-related fatigue in women undergoing adjuvant therapy for breast cancer. *J. Clin. Oncol.*, 23, 27, 6613-6622.

Anisman, H., Baines, M.G., Berczi, I., Bernstein, C.N., Blennerhassett, M.G., Gorczynski, R.M, et al. (1992) Neuroimmune mechanisms in health and disease: 2. Disease. *Can. Med. Assoc. J.*, 155, 1075-1092.

Beam, E. & Richardson, (1996) A. Fatigue: a concept analysis. *Int. J. Nurs. Stud.* 33, 519-529.

Berger, A. M. (1998) Patterns of fatigue and activity and rest during adjuvant breast cancer chemotherapy. *Oncol. Nurs. Forum,* 25, 51-62.

Bilbo, S.D., & Schwartz, T.N. (2009) Early-life programming of later-life brain and behavior: a critical role for the immune system. *Front Behav. Neurosci.*, 3, 14.

Blackwell, T.S. & Christman, J.W. (1996) Sepsis and cytokines: current status. *Br J Anaesth* 77, 110-117.

Bower J.E., Ganz P.A., Desmond K.A., Rowland J.H., Meyerowitz B.E., Belin, T.R. (2000) Fatigue in breast cancer survivors: occurrence, correlates, and impact on quality of life. *J. Clin. Oncol.*, 2000, 18, 743-753.

Bower, J.E., Ganz, P.A., Aziz, N., & Fahey, J.L. (2002) Fatigue and proinflammatory cytokine activity in breast cancer survivors. *Psychosom. Med.*, 64, 604-611.

Cella, D., Peterman, A., Paaski, S., Jacobsen,P.,& Breitbart.W. (1998) Progress towards guidelines for the manage-ment of fatigue. *Oncology,* 12, 364-377.

Chao, C.C., Janoff, E.N., Hu, S.X., Thomas, K., Gallagher, M., Tsang M., et al (1991). Altered cytokine release in peripheral blood mononuclear cell cultures from patients with the chronic fatigue syndrome. *Cytokines*, 3, 4, 292-298.

Curt, G. A., Breitbart, W., Cella, D., Groopman, J. E., Horning, S. J., Itri, L. M., Johnson, D. H., Miaskowski, C., Scherr, S. L., Portenoy, R. K. et al. (2000) Impact of cancer-related fatigue on the lives of patients: new findings from the Fatigue Coalition. *Oncologist*, 5, 353-360.

Demetri, G.D., Kris, M., Wade, J., Degos, L, & Cella, D. (1998) Quality-of-life benefit in chemotherapy patients treated with epoietin alfa is independent of disease response or tumor type: response from a prospective community oncology study. *J. Clin. Oncol.*, 16, 3412-3425.

Diaz, N., Menjon, S., Rolfo, C., Garcia-Alonso, P., Carulla, J., Magro, A., Miramon, J., Rodriguez, C. A., et al (2008) Patients' perception of cancer-related fatigue: results of a survey to assess the impact on their everyday life. *Clin. Transl. Oncol.*, 10, 753-757.

Dimeo, F., Schmittel, A., Fietz, T., Schwartz, S., Kohler, P., Boning, D. & Thiel, E. (2004) Physical performance, depression, immune status and fatigue in patients with hematological malignancies after treatment. *Ann. Oncol.*, 2004, 15, 1237-1242.

Geinitz, H., Zimmermann, F.B., Stoll, P., & Thamm, R., Kaffenberger, W., Ansorg, K., et al. (2001) Fatigue, serum cytokine levels, and blood cell counts during radiotherapy of patients with breast cancer. *Int. J. Radiat. Oncol. Biol. Phys.*, 51, 3, 691-698.

Glaus, A., Crow, R. & Hammond, S. A (1996) qualitative study to explore the concept of fatigue/tiredness in cancer patients and in healthy individuals. *Support. Care Cancer*, 4, 2, 82-96.

Glasby, J., Bukowski, J.R., Steinberg, D., Taylor, C., Tchekmedyian, S., & Vadhan-Raj, S. (1997) Impact of therapy with epoetin alfa on clinical outcomes in patients with non-myeloid malignancies during cancer chemotherapy in community oncology practise. *J. Clin. Oncol.*, 15, 1218-1234.

Gutstein, H. B. (2001) The biologic basis of fatigue. *Cancer*, 92, 1678 -1683.

Hann, D.M., Jacobsen, P.B., Azzarello, L.M., Martin, S.C., Curran, S.L., Fields, K.K. et al. (1988) Measurement of fatigue in cancer patients: development and validation of the Fatigue Symptom Inventory. *Qual. Life Res.*, 7, 301-310.

Hartvig, P., Aulin, J., Hugerth, M., Wallenberg, S. & Wagenius, G. (2006a) Fatigue in cancer patients treated with chemotherapy drugs. *J. Oncol. Pharm.* Pract., 12, 155-164.

Hartvig, P., Aulin, J., Wallenberg, S. & Wagenius, G. (2006b) Physical exercise for chemotherapy drug-induced fatigue. *J. Oncol. Pharm. Pract.*, 12, 183-191.

Hartvig-Honoré, P. (2010) Fatigue - a challenging symptom for cancer patients treated with cytotoxic drugs – mechanisms and targets for treatment. *Ann. Pharmaceut. Franc.*, 68, 76 -81.

Hong, J.H., Chiang, C.S., Campbell, I.L, Sun, J.R., Withers, H.R.& McBride WH. (1993) Induction of acute phase gene expression by brain irradiation. *Int. J. Radiat. Oncol. Biol. Phys.*, 33, 3, 619-624.

Hwang, S. S., Chang, V. T., Rue, M. and Kasimis, B. (2003) Multidimensional independent predictors of cancer-related fatigue. *J. Pain Symptom. Manage.*, 26, 1, 604-614.

Irvine, D., Vincent, L., Graydon, J., Bubela, N., & Thompson, L. (1994) The prevalence and correlates of fatigue in patients receiving treatment with chemotherapyc drugs and radiotherapy. *Cancer Nurs.*, 17, 367-378.

Jacobsen, P. B., Hann, D. M., Azzarello, L. M., Horton, J., Balducci, L.& Lyman, G. H. (1999) Fatigue in women receiving adjuvant chemotherapy for breast cancer: characteristics, course, and correlates.*J. Pain Symptom Managem.*, 199, 18, 233-242.

Jacobsen, P. B., Donovan, K. A., Small, B. J., Jim, H. S., Munster, P. N. & Andrykowski, M. A. (2007) Fatigue after treatment for early stage breast cancer: a controlled comparison. *Cancer*, 110, 1851-1859.

Jong, D.N., Candel, M.J., Schouten, H.C., Abu-Saad, H.H. & Courtens, A.M. (2004) Prevalence and course of fatigue in breast cancer patients receiving adjuvant chemotherapy. *Ann. Oncol.*, 15, 896-905.

Kalman D. Nutritional aspects of cancer-related fatigue. *J Am Diet Assoc* 1997, 97, 650-654.

Kim, S. H., Son, B. H., Hwang, S. Y., Han, W., Yang, J. H., Lee, S. and Yun, Y. H.(2008) Fatigue and depression in disease-free breast cancer survivors: prevalence, correlates, and association with quality of life. *J. Pain Symptom Managem.*, 35, 6, 644-655.

Kurzrock, R. (2001) The role of cytokines in cancer-related fatigue. *Cancer*, 92, 1684-1688.

Larisch, R., Klimke, A., Mayoral, F., Hamacher, K., Herzog, H.R., Vosberg, H. et al. (2001) Disturbance of serotonin 5HT2 receptors in remitted patients suffering from hereditary depressive disorder. *Nuklearmedizin*, 40, 4, 4, 19-34.

Liu, L., Fiorentino, L., Natarajan, L., Parker, B. A., Mills, P. J., Sadler, G. R., Dimsdale, J. E., Rissling, M., He, F. & Ancoli-Israel, S. (2009) Pre-treatment symptom cluster in breast cancer patients is associated with worse sleep, fatigue and depression during chemotherapy. *Psycho-Oncology,* 18, 187 - 194.

Mamounas, L.A., Altar, C,A., Blue, M.E., Kaplan, D.R., Tessarollo, L, & Lyons, W.E. (2000) BDNF promotes the regenerative sprouting, but not survival, of injured serotonergic axons in the adult rat brain. *J. Neurosci.*, 20, 771 - 782.

Midtgaard, J., Baadsgaard, M. T., Moller, T., Rasmussen, B., Quist, M., Andersen, C., Rorth, M. & Adamsen, L. (2009) Self-reported physical activity behavior; exercise motivation and information among Danish adult cancer patients undergoing chemotherapy. *Eur. J. Oncol. Nurs.*, 13, 116-121.

Mock, V., Atkinson, A., Barsevick, A., Cella, D., Cimprich, B., Cleeland, C., Donnelly, J., Eisenberger, M. A., Escalante, C., Hinds, P. et al. (2000) NCCN Practice Guidelines for Cancer-Related Fatigue. *Oncology,* 1, 151-161.

Morrow, G.R., Andrews, P.L., Hickok, J.T, Roscoe, J.A., & Matteson., S. (2002) Fatigue associated with cancer and its treatment. *Support. Care Cancer,* 10, 389-398.

Nitta, A., Ito, M., Fukumitsu, H., Ohmiya, M., Ito, H., Sometani, A., Nomoto, H, et al. (1994) 4-methylcatechol increases brain-derived neurotrophic factor content and mRNA expression in cultured brain cells and in rat brain in vivo. *J. Pharmacol. Exp. Ther.*, 291, 1276 - 83.

O´Donnel, J.F., Insomnia in cancer patients. *Clinical cornerstone,* 2004, Vol 6, Suppl 1D, S6-14.

Pater, J.L., Zee, B., Palmer, M., Johnston, S., & Osoba,D. (1997) Fatigue in patients with cancer:results from National Cancer Institute of Canada clinical trial group studies employing EORTC-QLQ-C30. *Support Cancer Care,* 5, 410 - 413.

Patrick, D.L., Ferketich, S.L., Frame, P.S., Harris, J.J., Hendricks, C.B., Levin, B, et al. (2002) National Institutes of Health State-of-the-Science Conference Statement: Symptom management in cancer: Pain, depression, and fatigue, July 15-17, 2002. *J. National Cancer Institute,* 95 (15), 1110-1117.

Piper, B.F., Lindsey, A.M., & Dodd, M. (1987) Fatigue mechanisms in cancer patients: Developing nursing theory. *Oncol. Nurs. Forum,* 14, 6, 17-23.

Piper, B. (1993) Fatigue and cancer inevitable companions *Support Care Cancer,* 1, 1286-1288.

Pud, D., Ben, A.S., Cooper, B. A., Aouizerat, B. E., Cohen, D., Radiano, R., Naveh, P., Nikkhou-Abeles, R., Hagbi, V., Kachta, O. et al. (2008) The symptom experience of oncology outpatients has a different impact on quality-of-life outcomes. *J. Pain Symptom. Managem.*, 35, 162-170.

Ream, E. & Richardson, A. (1996) Fatigue: a concept analysis. *Int. J. Nurs. Stud.*, 33, 519-529.

Ream, E. & Richardson,A. (1997) Fatigue in patients with cancer and chronic obstructive airways disease: a phenomenological enquiry. *Int. J. Nurs. Stud.*, 34, 1, 44-53.

Redeker, N. S., Lev, E. L. & Ruggiero, J. (2000) Insomnia, fatigue, anxiety, depression, and quality of life of cancer patients undergoing chemotherapy. *Sch. Inq. Nurs. Pract.*, 14, 275 - 290

Richardson, A.(1995) Fatigue in cancer patients Review of the literature. *Eur. J. Cancer Care,* 4, 20-28.

Richardson, A., Ream, E., & Wilson-Barnett, J. (1998) Fatigue in patients receiving chemotherapy patterns of change. *Cancer Nursing,* 21, 17-30.

Romito, F., Montanaro, R., Corvasce, C., Di, B. M. & Mattioli, V. (2008) Is cancer-related fatigue more strongly correlated to hematological or to psychological factors in cancer patients? *Support. Care Cancer,* 16, 943-946.

Rosel, P., Arranz, B., San, L., Vallejo, J., Crespo, J.M., Urretavizcaya, M, et al. (2000) Altered 5-HT(2A) binding sites and second messenger inositol trisphosphate (IP(3)) levels in hippocampus but not in frontal cortex from depressed suicide victims. *Psychiatry Res.*, 99, 173 -81.

Rumajogee, P., Madeira, A., Verge, D,, Hamon, M., & Miquel, M.C. (2002) Up-regulation of the neuronal serotoninergic phenotype in vitro: BDNF and cAMP share Trk B-dependent mechanisms. *J. Neurochem.*, 83, 1525-1528.

Sapolsky, R.M., Uno, H., Rebert, C.S., Finch, C.E, et al. (1990) Hippocampal damage associated with prolonged glucocorticoid exposure in primates. *J. Neurosci.*, 10, 2897-2902.

Schwartz.,A. (2000) Daily Fatigue patterns and effect of exercise in women with breast cancer. *Cancer Practice*, 8(1), 16-24.

Shirayama, Y., Chen, A.C, Nakagawa, S., Russell, D.S., Duman, R.S..(2002) Brain-derived neurotrophic factor produces antidepressant effects in behavioral models of depression. *J. Neurosci.*, 22, 3251-61.

Steensberg, A., Fisher, C.P., Keller, C., Moller, K., & Pedersen, B.K. (2006) Il-6 increases IL-1ra, IL-10 and cortisol in humans *Am. J. Physiol. Endocrinol. Metab.*, 285, E434 -E437.

Stockmeier, C.A. (2003) Involvement of serotonin in depression: evidence from postmortem and imaging studies of serotonin receptors and the serotonin transporter. *J Psychiatr. Res.*, 37, 357-73.

Swain, G. (2000) Fatigue in chronic disease. *Clin. Sci.*, 99, 1-8.

Tartaglia, L.A., & Goeddel, D.V. (1992) Two TNF receptors. *Immunol. Today.* 13, 151-153.

van Loon, G.R., Shum, A., & Sole, M.J. (1981) Decreased brain serotonin turnover after short term (two-hour) adrenalectomy in rats: a comparison of four turnover methods. *Endocrinology*, 108, 1392 - 402.

Watanabe, A., Tohyama, Y., Nguyen, K.Q., Hasegawa, S., Debonnel, G., Diksic, M., et al. (2003) Regional brain serotonin synthesis is increased in the olfactory bulbectomy rat model of depression: an autoradiographic study. *J. Neurochem.*, 85, 469-75.

Wilson, A., Hickie, I., Lloyd, A., Hadzi-Pavlovic, D., Boughton, C., Dwyer, J. & Wakefield, D. (1994) Longitudinal study of outcome of chronic fatigue syndrome. *Brit. Med. J.*, , 308, 756-759.

Yamagishi, A., Morita, T., Miyashita, M. & Kimura, F. (2009) Symptom prevalence and longitudinal follow-up in cancer outpatients receiving chemotherapy. *J. Pain Symtom. Managem.*, 37, 5, 823-830.

Yennurajalingam, S., Palmer, J. L., Zhang, T., Poulter, V. & Bruera, E. (2008). Association between fatigue and other cancer-related symptoms in patients with advanced cancer. *Support Care Cancer*, 16, 1125-1130.

5

The Diagnosis and Treatment of Insomnia

Michał Skalski
Department of Psychiatry Medical University of Warsaw,
Sleep Disorders Outpatients Clinic
Poland

1. Introduction

Insomnia is the most common sleep disorder. It is also, together with pain and fatigue, the most common ailment among all of us. Insomnia can be a standalone diagnostic category, but just like fever or pain, can be a symptom of another disease, either somatic or mental. Though insomnia is a prevalent condition in our society, both doctors and patients are lacking in the knowledge about it. There are also no generally accepted standards of treatment, especially the pharmacological.

Sleepless nights happen to everyone. Many scientists and most of the society think of insomnia as a natural reaction of the organism to tension or noise. The popular opinion is right. It is natural - this condition is called short-term insomnia or adjustment insomnia (according to ICSD – International Classification of Sleep Disorders; AASM, 2005) - when the sleeplessness is related to stress and anxiety. But as the researches show - the short-term insomnia can easily transform into a chronic condition. Numerous epidemiological studies have discovered that about 30% of the world's population, including more than 50% of people older than 60 and almost 20% of those younger declare sleep disorders. One third of these cases can be qualified as chronic insomnia (Ohayan, 1997; Szelenberger & Skalski 1999).

There are many explanations of such a distinctive increase in number of complaints of insomnia, as the natural adjustment to the changing world, lifestyle, circadian rhythm disorders or as a syndrome of worsening physical and mental state of society. Although some facts are hard to disagree with, it is worth to mention that some researchers say it does not make much sense to talk about insomnia in the categories we got used to. They believe sleep is just one of our basic needs - we sleep to deal with fatigue as we eat to deal with hunger. They compare insomnia to obesity - both result from an inappropriate lifestyle. Eating too much results in obesity. Being lazy and having exaggerated expectations of the sleep result in insomnia. Authors of these ideas underpin their concepts with researches of animals' sleep where the animals living in natural conditions having to fight for their survival sleep distinctively shorter than the ones living in safety of a laboratory. In conclusion, we complain of insomnia because we are wealthy, safe and have too much spare time we want to fill with sleeping (Anderson & Horne, 2008).

Can the modern science help us to resolve these dilemmas? In the following book chapter we will try to resolve problems associated with diagnosing and treating insomnia and will try to present practical solutions for sleeplessness.

2. Insomnia - definitions, diagnostic criteria

What is insomnia? A basic definition of insomnia can be easily derived from what we have describe before. Insomnia is a subjective feeling of not getting enough sleep in terms of its length and quality together with its consequences, such as being unproductive and in bad mood during daytime.

Types of insomnia:

Insomnia is generally divided into primary and secondary insomnia. Primary insomnia appears for no apparent reason, secondary is related to another diseases. Another popular criteria are how long insomnia persists. Transient insomnia lasts for a few days to a week, acute insomnia (up to one month) and chronic insomnia (more than one month) (NIMH, 1984).

2.1 Criteria of diagnosing insomnia

The following are the most common and accepted definitions and diagnostic criteria of insomnia according to ICD-10, DSM-IV-TR and ICSD-2, (WHO 1992; APA, 2000; AASM, 2005).

ICD-10 diagnosis code F51 (WHO, 1992)

Sleep disorders not due to a substance or known physiological condition

F51.0 Nonorganic insomnia. A condition of unsatisfactory quantity and/or quality of sleep, which persists for a considerable period of time, including difficulty falling asleep, difficulty staying asleep, or early final wakening. Insomnia is a common symptom of many mental and physical disorders, and should be classified here in addition to the basic disorder only if it dominates the clinical picture. Excludes: insomnia (organic) (G47.0)

ICD-10 diagnosis code G47 (WHO, 1992)

Sleep disorders

G47.0 Disorders of initiating and maintaining sleep [insomnias]

ICD-10 diagnostic criteria for non-organic insomnia

a. A complaint of excessive daytime sleepiness or sleep attacks or prolonged transition to the fully aroused state upon awakening (sleep drunkenness) (not accounted for by an inadequate amount of sleep).
b. This sleep disturbance occurs nearly every day for at least one month or recurrently for shorter periods of time and either causes marked distress or interference with personal functioning in daily living.
c. Absence of auxiliary symptoms of narcolepsy (cataplexy, sleep paralysis, hypnagogic hallucinations) or of clinical evidence for sleep apnea (nocturnal breath cessation, typical intermittent snorting sounds, etc.).

d. Absence of any known causative organic factor, such as a neurological or other medical condition, psychoactive substance use disorder or a medication.

DSM-IV-TR diagnostic criteria for primary insomnia (APA, 2000)

a. The predominant complaint is difficulty initiating or maintaining sleep, or nonrestorative sleep, for at least 1 month.
b. The sleep disturbance (or associated daytime fatigue) causes clinically significant distress
c. The sleep disturbance does not occur exclusively during the course of narcolepsy, breathing-related sleep disorder, circadian rhythm sleep disorder, or parasomnia.
d. The disturbance does not occur exclusively during the course of another mental disorder (e.g., major depressive disorder, generalized anxiety disorder, a delirium).
e. The disturbance is not due to the direct physiological effects of a substance.

Diagnostic criteria for insomnia (ICSD-2, 2005)

a. A complaint of difficulty initiating sleep, difficulty maintaining sleep, or waking up too early, or sleep that is chronically nonrestorative or poor in quality.
b. The above sleep difficulty occurs despite adequate opportunity and circumstances for sleep.
c. At least one of the following forms of daytime impairment related to the nighttime sleep difficulty is reported by the patient:
    1. Fatigue or malaise;
    2. Attention, concentration, or memory impairment;
    3. Social or vocational dysfunction or poor school performance;
    4. Mood disturbance or irritability;
    5. Daytime sleepiness;
    6. Motivation, energy, or initiative reduction;
    7. Proneness for errors/accidents at work or while driving;
    8. Tension, headaches, or gastrointestinal symptoms in response to sleep loss; and
    9. Concerns or worries about sleep.

In conclusion, according to the diagnostic criteria listed above, we need the following symptoms to diagnose insomnia:

1. Presence of sleep disorders (difficulty falling asleep, difficulty staying asleep, or early wakening) during the better part of the night and persistent for at least one month
2. Worsened daytime functioning caused by these sleep disorders.

ICD-10 classifications also divide insomnia into different forms

ICD-10 sleep disorders

- organic insomnia
- nonorganic insomnia

DSM-IV diagnoses of sleep disorders

- Primary sleep disorders
- Dyssomnias
- Primary insomnia

- Sleep disorders related to another mental disorder
- Insomnia related to another mental disorder
- Secondary sleep disorders due to an Axis III condition
- Insomnia type
- Substance-induced sleep disorders
- Insomnia type

ICSD-2 sleep disorder categories - insomnias (specific disorders)

Adjustment (acute) insomnia

The essential feature of this disorder is the presence of insomnia in association with an identifiable stressor, such as psychosocial, physical, or environmental disturbances. The sleep disturbance has a relatively short duration (days-weeks) and is expected to resolve when the stressor resolves.

Psychophysiological insomnia

The essential features of this disorder are heightened arousal and learned sleep-preventing associations. Arousal may be physiological, cognitive, or emotional, and characterized by muscle tension, "racing thoughts," or heightened awareness of the environment. Individuals typically have increased concern about sleep difficulties and their consequences, leading to a "vicious cycle" of arousal, poor sleep, and frustration.

Paradoxical insomnia

The essential feature of this disorder is a complaint of severe or nearly "total" insomnia that greatly exceeds objective evidence of sleep disturbance and is not commensurate with the reported degree of daytime deficit. Although paradoxical insomnia is best diagnosed with concurrent PSG and self-reports, it can be presumptively diagnosed on clinical grounds alone. To some extent, "misperception" of the severity of sleep disturbance may characterize all insomnia disorders.

Idiopathic insomnia

The essential feature of this disorder is a persistent complaint of insomnia with insidious onset during infancy or early childhood and no or few extended periods of sustained remission. Idiopathic insomnia is not associated with specific precipitating or perpetuating factors.

Insomnia due to mental disorder

The essential feature of this disorder is the occurrence of insomnia that occurs exclusively during the course of a mental disorder, and is judged to be caused by that disorder. The insomnia is of sufficient severity to cause distress or to require separate treatment. This diagnosis is not used to explain insomnia that has a course independent of the associated mental disorder, as is not routinely made in individuals with the "usual" severity of sleep symptoms for an associated mental disorder.

Inadequate sleep hygiene

The essential feature of this disorder is insomnia associated with voluntary sleep practices or activities that are inconsistent with good sleep quality and daytime alertness. These practices and activities typically produce increased arousal or directly interfere with sleep, and may include irregular sleep scheduling, use of alcohol, caffeine, or nicotine, or engaging in non-sleep behaviors in the sleep environment. Some element of poor sleep hygiene may characterize individuals with other insomnia disorders.

Insomnia due to a drug or substance

The essential feature of this disorder is sleep disruption due to use of a prescription medication, recreational drug, caffeine, alcohol, food, or environmental toxin. Insomnia may occur during periods of use/exposure, or during discontinuation. When the identified substance is stopped, and after discontinuation effects subside, the insomnia is expected to resolve or substantially improve.

Insomnia due to medical condition

The essential feature of this disorder is insomnia caused by a coexisting medical disorder or other physiological factor. Although insomnia is commonly associated with many medical conditions, this diagnosis should be used when the insomnia causes marked distress or warrants separate clinical attention. This diagnosis is not used to explain insomnia that has a course independent of the associated medical disorder, and is not routinely made in individuals with the "usual" severity of sleep symptoms for an associated medical disorder.

Insomnia not due to substance or known physiologic condition, unspecified; physiologic (organic) insomnia, unspecified

These two diagnoses are used for insomnia disorders that cannot be classified elsewhere but are suspected to be related to underlying mental disorders, psychological factors, behaviors, medical disorders, physiological states, or substance use or exposure. These diagnoses are typically used when further evaluation is required to identify specific associated conditions, or when the patient fails to meet criteria for a more specific disorder.

Judging the categories presented above from a practical and clinical point of view we have to admit that none of them is sufficient for diagnosing and treatment of insomnia. ICD-10 divides insomnia into nonorganic and organic form which is a big simplification while ICSD proposes a way too complicated categorizing which does not make it useful in everyday practice. Definitely, the most useful of all systems is the DSM-IV-TR classification system, dividing insomnia into 4 categories:

- Primary insomnia
- Insomnia related to another mental disorder
- Insomnia due to medical disorders
- Substance-induced insomnia

We estimate that this classification is the most useful and helpful in diagnosis and treatment of insomnia.

2.2 Practical categorization of insomnia

Because other chapters of this book encompasses a complex analysis of secondary insomnia, in the following part we are going to focus on the pure-form primary insomnia, described also as nonorganic insomnia, primary insomnia or psychophysiological insomnia in different diagnostic criteria. When diagnosing a new patient it is very important to properly assess the problem. We have to know if the troubles a patient declares meet criteria of insomnia. Based on carefully collected medical history about behaviors related to sleep and sleep diary analysis we often see that many patients, especially the older ones, spend 8 to 10 hours daily in bed, sleeping only 5 to 7 hours in that time. As a result, though they sleep well, their time spent in bed includes a few additional hours of WASO (Wakefulness After Sleep Onset). Such a state can hardly be classified as a real insomnia; though a patient does not fulfill their entire need for sleep, it has to be said that patient's expectations of sleeping through 8 hours in the night without interruptions are not realistic. Sleep disorder like this cannot be classified as insomnia; we can call them inadequate sleep hygiene or unrealistic expectations of sleep. Treatment of these disorders should not be done by fulfilling patient's expectations, but by making them more realistic. A second group of sleep disorders often wrongly classified as insomnia concerns mainly young people complaining about sleepiness during daytime, fatigue and troubles with waking up in the morning. But the analysis of their behaviour and sleep diary shows that usually because of work, learning or play almost every night they sleep less than other in the same age group. Such a state called sleep deprivation rather not insomnia.

After diagnosing the real insomnia, the most important part is determining how long it persists. The traditional categorizing divides insomnia into:

- Transient insomnia - a few days
- Acute insomnia - up to 4 weeks
- Chronic insomnia - longer than one month (NIMH, 1984).

Transient insomnia lasts for a few days to a week, acute insomnia (up to one month) and chronic insomnia (more than one month). Transient and acute insomnias are usually related to some kind of trigger (stress, noise, pain). Chronic insomnia can be related to another sickness but more often, it is caused by so - called perpetuating factors which cause insomnia to remain even when the primary causation of it is gone. We can conclude that while the short-term insomnia is usually secondary, the chronic one becomes primary.

2.3 Insomnia diagnosis

Because only 1 / 3 of patients reported their sleep problems to physician (Szelenberger & Skalski, 1999, Pentor 2000), undoubtedly the first and most important task in the diagnostic process is to find patients with sleep disorders. It is therefore recommended that the questions about the quality of sleep and mood in the morning are a regular part of every medical interview, in almost every medical specialty. Patients with insomnia should go immediately to their general practitioners and begin the correct treatment.

The main diagnostic tool is the interview focused on sleep, respectively, accompanied by any further diagnostic tests for determining somatic or psychiatric causes of insomnia (Table 1).

2.4 Development of chronic insomnia

Modern views on etiology and pathogenesis of insomnia show correlation between various biological, medical and environmental factors in creating insomnia and causing it to persist. These factors can be divided into 3 groups – 3P (Spielman, 1986):

Predisposing factors - being prone to insomnia, biological grounds like personality, maintaining circadian rhythm, age, genetics.

I. Interview schedule:
1st Determine the type and nature of sleep disorders:
2nd Disease and associated factors:
- Somatic diseases and medications - Psychosocial stress - Mood disorders
3rd Sleep before the onset of symptoms:
- The quality of sleep before the onset of insomnia - The earlier episodes of insomnia - Other sleep disorders - Reaction to treatment
4th Sleep hygiene:
- Time of lie down and getting up from bed - Sleep on weekdays and holidays - Variable working hours in the day and night, shift work - Naps during the day - Physical exercise habits and lifestyle - Consumption of coffee, alcohol and other drugs
5th Information from bed partner:
- Snoring and irregular breathing - Movements during sleep - Evaluation of sleep length and quality of patient - Changes in mood and behavior of the patient
II. Somatic Research, depending on the patient's complaints focused on the search:
1st rheumatic
2nd respiratory and ENT
3rd cardiovascular
4th renal
5th neurological
6th cancer
7th gastrological
III. Psychiatric and psychological assessment:
1st on the basis of conversation
- Behavior changes
- Mood changes
- Anxiety
- Psychosocial stress situations
- Excessive preoccupation with his dream
2nd based on scales, e.g.
- Beck Depression Scale (self) - Hamilton Depression Rating Scale - Hamilton anxiety scale - Dementia assessment scale (Mini Mental State) - MMPI personality assessment scale

3rd eventual referral to a psychologist or psychiatrist
IV. Sleep monitoring studies:
1st polysomnographic study
2nd actigraphic registration
3rd study MSLT (Multiple Sleep Latency Test allows an objective assessment of excessive sleepiness)

Table 1. Examination scheme of patients with sleep disorders

Precipitating (Triggers) factors causing sleep interruptions directly - environmental, adaptive, medical

Perpetuating factors - drugs abuse, improper sleep hygiene, exaggerated expectations of sleep, the fear of insomnia - often create a vicious circle of insomnia.

There is more and more evidence that people with insomnia are constantly in the state of so-called hyperarousal. Many of them are less sleepy during daytime, which can be measured by studying duration of their naps. These people also have significantly increased metabolism level during the whole 24 hours. Consequently, assumptions have been made that in patients with chronic insomnia the main and most common problem is the excessive arousal responsible both for poor functioning during daytime and problems with sleep at night. People with insomnia have increased ACTH level and raised cortisol secretion and lowered inhibitory neurotransmitter GABA level. (Bonnet & Arand, 1997; Perlis et al. 1998; Vgontzas et al. 1998; Winkelman et al., 2008)

Knowledge of the mechanisms listed above is extremely important for successful treatment requiring focus on various aspects of insomnia. Contemporary rules say that the treatment should be commenced with the occurrence of the very first symptoms of insomnia to quickly eliminate the causes and avoid perpetuating mechanisms.

3. Treatment of insomnia

When to start with treatment of insomnia, how and by whom should it be treated?

In any case, if sleep problems persist for longer than 2-3 weeks and begin to negatively impact on functioning during the day, be sure to seek medical advice.

In the case of short-term insomnia, especially in those predisposed to insomnia, it is necessary to take treatment as soon as possible. It is usually sufficient administration of temporary hypnotic drug. The patient places the sleeping pill, near the bed and reaches for it when can not sleep. This treatment protects the patient against the occurrence of factors perpetuate insomnia and prevents against the development of chronic insomnia.

In chronic insomnia administration of hypnotics is neither effective nor consistent with the principles of administration of hypnotics (no longer than 2-4 weeks). In addition, perpetuates and worsening course of insomnia and increases the risk of dependence on hypnotics. The primary method of treatment for chronic insomnia is behavioral therapy.

3.1 Non-pharmacological treatment of insomnia

There are numerous methods of non-pharmacological treatment of insomnia. They include:

- - information on the sleep hygiene principles,
- - stimulus control,
- - sleep restriction,
- - relaxation techniques,
- - feedback,
- - cognitive therapy,
- - "chronotherapy",
- - phytotherapy (Morin, 1999; Yang, 2005; Schutte-Rodin, 2008).

3.1.1 Behavioral techniques

3.1.1.1 Sleep hygiene education

The sleep hygiene principles include: refraining from naps during the day; getting to sleep and getting up at the same time; restraining or giving up consumption of caffeine, alcohol and nicotine; avoiding physical activities shortly before moving to bed, staying away of any emotional arousal before bedtime, ensuring quiet environment and comfortable temperature in a bedroom, removing clocks from a bedroom (Hauri & Fisher, 1986).

3.1.1.2 Sleep restriction

A sleep restriction means for the patient being in bed no longer than usually sleeps at night, according to his subjective assessment (for example, by sleep diary). As the sleep's length is usually underestimated, the patient will partially deprive his sleep, reducing at the same time the number of awakenings the following night (Spielmann et al. 1987).

3.1.1.3 Stimulus control therapy

Stimulus control technique aims to restrict the bedroom and the bed for a sleep only. Reading, eating and watching television in bed is prohibited. The patient should go to bed only when feeling sleepy. If a sleep does not come within the next ten minutes, he has to get up, go to another room and return only when feeling sleepy. An alarm clock should be set always at the same time, regardless of a sleep's length. The patient also has to refrain from naps during the day (Bootzin et al. 1991).

3.1.2 Cognitive therapy

Insomnia-related concerns increase insomnia, causing excitation and further exacerbate sleep problems. It has been proven that the erroneous beliefs and attitudes toward sleep are associated with symptoms of insomnia. Changing negative thoughts can reduce concerns about the lack of sleep and break the vicious circle leading to excitation and insomnia.

Common incorrect beliefs about sleep can be classified into five categories:

1. misunderstanding of insomnia's causes,
2. seeking incorrect or exaggerated insomnia consequences
3. unrealistic expectations of sleep,

4. limited perception of control over sleep
5. belief that sleep could be predictable.

Incorrect beliefs about sleep can be corrected by educating patients about the principles of the sleep hygiene. The aim of the cognitive therapy is the recognition by the patient that he can cope with the problem of insomnia. (Morin et al. 1999; 2002).

For several years, in Warsaw Sleep Disorders Clinic we regularly conduct CBT group therapy (six sessions, every week, number of patients 6-10). Our findings confirmed the high efficacy of the CBT therapy. CBT-I produced sustained self-reported improvement in nocturnal sleep and daytime functioning (Fornal-Pawłowska et al., 2010). After 3 months, insomniacs did not differ from good sleepers in sleep quality and social functioning ratings (Fig. 1 and 2).

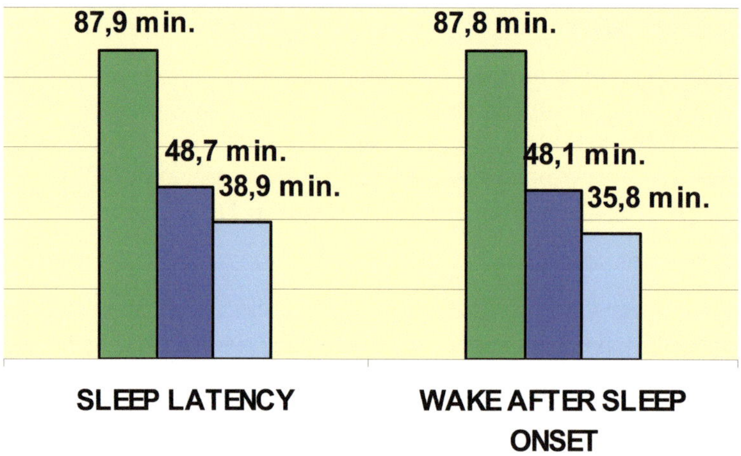

Fig. 1. Changes in sleep parameters: sleep latency and WASO, at baseline, post-treatment and the 3-month follow-up

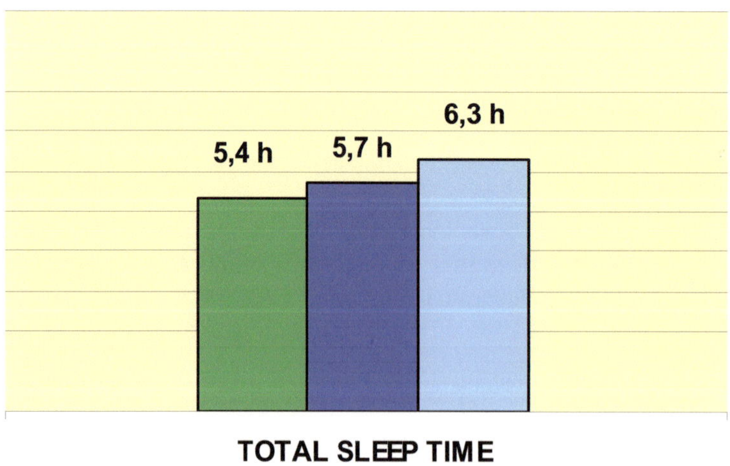

Fig. 2. Changes in total sleep time at baseline, post-treatment and the 3-month follow-up

3.1.3 Summary of non-pharmacologic strategies

For the past 10 years in our sleep disorders clinic in Warsaw CBT of insomnia has become a routine method of treatment for chronic insomnia. It consists of 6 sessions which take place once a week, in groups consisting of 6-10 people. In the following sessions, patients are educated about the physiology of sleep and sleep disorders. Then learn the next technique: education about sleep hygiene, sleep restriction, stimulus control, relaxation exercises, and finally cognitive therapy oriented at dysfunctional thoughts related to insomnia. In parallel, patients receive information about rational pharmacotherapy of insomnia, which is only occasional use of hypnotics (2-3 times a week) and possibly the use of low doses of antidepressant drugs or herbal medicines. The results so far are very promising (shown in the Figures above) and indicate that the CBT treatment of insomnia is currently the most effective treatment for chronic insomnia.

3.2 Pharmacological treatment of insomnia

Drug treatment is indicated for patients as short-term relief of symptoms of insomnia but is insufficient for long-term management of chronic insomnia. In combination with cognitive-behavioral therapy, it gives the best results in improving the quality of sleep. (Riemann&Perlis, 2009; Saddichha, 2010).

3.2.1 Benzodiazepine Receptor Agonists (BZD or newer BzRAs)

The most widely used method for insomnia is to administer benzodiazepine receptor agonists (Yang, 2005; Schutte-Rodin, 2008). This group includes all the traditional benzodiazepines (BZD) and hypnotics new generation (benzodiazepine receptor agonists - BzRAs) - zolpidem, zopiclone and zaleplon.

3.2.1.1 Benzodiazepines

The selection of a specific benzodiazepine agonist should be performed in accordance with the knowledge of its pharmacokinetics. When changing the medication, be sure to equivalent doses of different preparations.

Objective results of treatment with hypnotics are small: latency is shortened by 15 minutes and total sleep time increased by about 30 minutes. Benzodiazepines do not improve sleep quality. Rapidly lose their hypnotic effect, sometimes after a few days. Dependence develops after regular ingestion of several weeks. Prevention of tolerance and addiction is the administration of hypnotics no more than 2-3 times a week and the lowest dose, repeat the drug at intervals of less than four times the value of its half-life leading to accumulation (Walsh et al. 2000; Hajak et al. 2002; Perlis, 2004).

3.2.1.2 Non-benzodiazepine hypnotics

In comparison with traditional BZD new generation hypnotic drugs appear to be a major step forward. Zolpidem and zaleplon are selective benzodiazepines receptor agonist. Because of their selective action on the omega-1 receptor, subclass of BZD receptors they do not affect cognition, memory and motor function. Zolpidem, zopiclone, and zaleplon rapidly absorbed and have a short biological half-life. This is important because residual symptoms the next day, that is, impairment of psychomotor skills and memory, depend on the biological half-life time. It is believed that the new benzodiazepine receptor agonists hypnotics give less risk of tolerance and dependence.

Need to be aware that in a patient with insomnia, hypnotic drug administration is only supportive care, relieving symptom of disease rather than treating disease.

Of course, the effects of hypnotics may be helpful in the general treatment of insomnia, when once again "we teach" patients sleep. But leaving the patient without the comprehensive support reduces the effectiveness of treatment, and very easily lead to addiction

3.2.2 Summarize the role of hypnotics in insomnia

In the short-term insomnia:

- Recognize as soon as possible insomnia and give patients a new generation of hypnotics (zolpidem, zopiclone, zaleplon), which may prevent in a patient developing in perpetuating factors
- The best method is to put the sleeping pills near the bed and reaching for it, when the patient is waiting too long to fall asleep after laying to bed, or in the event of the night awakenings
- Such way taking of sleeping pills will allow most patients with insomnia to avoid short-term transition in chronic insomnia, and at the same time protect them from dependence on hypnotics.
- The experiences of our everyday practice show that mere possession of an effective sleeping pills near the bed allows the patient to sleep better.

In the chronic insomnia:

- Do not chronic use of hypnotics (benzodiazepine receptor agonists), with daily use and must not be taken for more than 2 weeks.
- They can be take longer, but only if they are used temporarily "as needed" which is 2 to 3 times a week (or up to 10 times a month).
- Sleeping pills can be used if the patient also use behavioral techniques.
- Almost all patients after therapy, CBT, occasionally use sleeping pills, only a few times a month. Even if earlier abused benzodiazepines.

3.2.3 Sedative low dose antidepressant (AD)

In recent years, increasingly in the supportive treatment of insomnia is proposed to use the drugs from other groups deserve special attention and antidepressants, natural remedies, available without prescription (Thase, 1999; James & Mendelson 2004; Krystal et al. 2010).

In clinical practice, in case of necessity of prolonged treatment of insomnia alternative to the sleeping pills are antidepressants with sedative-hypnotic properties. The most commonly used drugs of such a profile are Trazodone, Mianserin, Mirtazapine, Doxepin. It has been proven that improves sleep in people suffering from insomnia and increases the amount of SWS. Some tricyclic antidepressants (TCAs) are also strong action sleeping pills. However, due to non-selective effect, causing more side effects.

There is no fixed standard dosage in the treatment of insomnia, usually are used in low doses in comparison to those used in depression. (James & Mendelson 2004; Krystal et al. 2010).

In everyday practice, Warsaw Sleep Disorders Clinic doses fully sufficient as a "hypnotic", are:

- mianserin 5 to 15 mg
- trazodone 25 do 100 mg
- mirtazapine 7,5 do 15 mg

The above mentioned dose are the smallest as possible to achieve (the tablets can not be divided any more), it is possible that even lower doses might be effective. Such small doses are usually very well tolerated and, in addition antidepressants do not give a risk of addiction. The most common side effect of what we find in our patients the symptoms of restless leg syndrome (RLS), usually after mianserin, less frequently after trazodone.

But even with such a small and safe doses should be avoided their chronic use, so that the patients do not used to falling asleep on the pills. Usually after a normalization of sleep and sleep hygiene correction also we recommend discontinuing medication.

3.2.4 Over-the-counter agents

In the insomnia is also used medicines available without prescription, such as melatonin, antihistamines and herbal medicines. These drugs are increasingly used (Montserrat Sanchez-Ortuno et al., 2009), but still is little systematic studies. From the few the available data it is estimated that natural remedies used from 4 to 18% of all people and from 30 to over 70% of those complaining of insomnia (Montserrat Sánchez-Ortuño et al., 2009; Sarris & Byrne, 2010; Salter & Brownie, 2010). So far performed too small amount of normal, placebo-controlled studies to evaluate the effectiveness of drugs used without a prescription for insomnia. Published in the last year review of all available studies of natural drugs and methods used in insomnia indicate an advantage of preparations containing valerian and hops in the improvement of various parameters of sleep (Montserrat Sánchez-Ortuño et al., 2009).

3.2.5 The risk of dependence

When discussing pharmacological treatment of insomnia can not ignore the problem dependence benzodiazepines. Experience our Sleep Disorders Clinic indicate that a large proportion of patients with chronic insomnia are more or less dependent on benzodiazepines. In a large part of patients, the existing dependence seems to be the primary cause of insomnia. In this case, the first stage of treatment is the gradual withdrawal of benzodiazepines and to manage the withdrawal symptoms. In the treatment of benzodiazepines dependence in patients with insomnia CBT therapy was very effective (Morin et al., 2004), also routinely used in our Warsaw Sleep Disorders Clinic.

4. Summary

The current rules establish that the treatment of insomnia should start right from the beginning of its occurrence, to avoid appearance of perpetuating factors - chronic insomnia development.

In the case of the diagnosis of transient or short-term insomnia, a basic method of treatment is usually administrating the right hypnotics and information on the sleep hygiene.

In chronic insomnia, a basic treatment is cognitive-behavioral therapy (CBT), which can help pharmacologically by regular use of "sedative and hypnotic" antidepressant medication in the evening only "as needed" taking hypnotics drugs (no more than 2-3 times a week).

5. References

American Academy of Sleep Medicine. (2005). *ICSD - International Classification of Sleep Disorders*, 2nd ed.: Diagnostic and coding manual. Westchester, Illinois: American Academy of Sleep Medicine.

American Psychiatric Association. (2000). *Diagnostic and Statistical Manual of Mental Disorders*, Fourth Edition, Text Revision. Washington, DC: The American Psychiatric Association; 2000.

Anderson C & Horne JA. (2008) Do we really want more sleep? A population-based study evaluating the strength of desire for more sleep. *Sleep Medicine,* 9, 184–187. ISSN: 1389-9457

Bixler E. (2009). Sleep and society: An epidemiological perspective. *Sleep Medicine, 10,* s3-s6. ISSN: 1389-9457

Bonnet MH, Arand DL. (1997). Hyperarousal and insomnia. *Sleep Med Rev.,* 2:97–108. ISSN: 1087-0792

Bootzin R.R., Epstain D., Wood J.M. (1991). Stimulus control instructions. In *Case Studies in Insomnia.* Hauri P. (ed.) Plenum Medical Book Co., New York. 19–28.

Borbely AA. (1982). A two process model of sleep regulation. *Hum Neurobiol.* 1, 195-204. ISSN: 0721-9075

Fornal-Pawlowska M., Skalski M., Szelenberger W. (2010). Cognitive behavioural therapy for insomnia. *Journal of Sleep Research* 2010; 19 (Suppl. 2): P479. 158

Hajak G, Cluydts R, Declerck A, Estivill SE, Middleton A, Sonka K, Unden M. (2002). Continuous versus non-nightly use of zolpidem in chronic insomnia: results of a large-scale, double-blind, randomized, outpatient study.*Int Clin Psychopharmacol.*(Jan) 17:9–17.

Hauri P., Fisher J. (1986). Persistent psychophysiologic (learned) insomnia. *Sleep.* 9: 38–53.

James SP, Mendelson WB. (2004). The use of trazodone as a hypnotic: a critical review. *J Clin Psychiatry.* 65:752–755. ISSN: 1555-2101

Kryger MH, Roth T & Dement C. (2011). *Principles and practice of sleep medicine.* 5th Edition. Elsevier Saunders Company, ISBN 978-1-4160-6645-3, Philadelphia.

Krystal AD; Durrence HH; Scharf M; Jochelson P; Rogowski R; Ludington E; Roth T. (2010). Efficacy and safety of doxepin 1 mg and 3 mg in a 12-week sleep laboratory and outpatient trial of elderly subjects with chronic primary insomnia. *Sleep,* 33(11). 1553-1561.

Montserrat Sánchez-Ortuño M ; Bélanger L; Ivers H; LeBlanc M; Morin CM. (2009). The use of natural products for sleep. A common practice? *Sleep Medicine.* 10. 982–987

Morin CM, Hauri PJ, Espie CA, Spielman AJ, Buysse DJ, Bootzin RR. (1999). Nonpharmacologic treatment of chronic insomnia. An American Academy of Sleep Medicine review. *Sleep,* 22:1–23.

Morin CM. (2002). Contributions of Cognitive-Behavioral Approaches to the Clinical Management of insomnia. *J Clin Psychiatry*, 4, suppl 1: 21-26

Morin CM, Bastien C, Guay B, Radouco-Thomas M, Leblanc J, Vallières A. (2004). Randomized Clinical Trial of Supervised Tapering and Cognitive Behavior Therapy to Facilitate Benzodiazepine Discontinuation in Older Adults With Chronic Insomnia. *Am J Psychiatry*; 161:332–342

National Institute of Mental Health. (1984). Drugs and Insomnia: The Use of Medications to Promote Sleep. *JAMA*. 251(18). 2410-2414. ISSN: 0098-7484

Ohayan MM, Caulet M, Priest RG, Guilleminault C. (1997). DSM-IV and ICSD-90 insomnia symptoms and sleep dissatisfaction. *Br J Psychiatry*, 171:382–388.

Pan-European Consumer Omnibus Study. (2000). Pentor.

Perlis ML, Giles DE, Mendelson WB, Bootzin RR, Wyatt JK. (1997). Psychophysiological insomnia: the behavioral model and a neurocognitive perspective. *J Sleep Res 1997*, 6:179–188. ISSN: 1365-2869

Perlis ML. (2004). Long-term, non-nightly administration of zolpidem in the treatment of patients with primary insomnia. *J Clin Psychiatry*.65:1128–37.

Riemann D, Perlis ML. (2009). The treatments of chronic insomnia: A review of benzodiazepine receptor agonists and psychological and behavioral therapies. *Sleep Med Rev*. 13: 205-14.

Saddichha S. (2010). Diagnosis and treatment of chronic insomnia. *Ann Indian Acad Neurol*. 21, 13: 94-102

Salter S; Brownie S. (2010). Treating primary insomnia - the efficacy of valerian and hops. *Australia in Family Physician*, 39, 6, june, 433-437

Saper CB, Chou TC, Scammell TE: (2001). The sleep switch: hypothalamic control of sleep and wakefulness. *Trends in Neurosciences*, 24, 12. 726-731. ISSN: 0166-2236

Saper CB, Lu J, Chou TC, Gooley J. (2005). The hypothalamic integrator for circadian rhythms. *Trends in Neurosciences*. 28, 3. 152–157. ISSN: 0166-2236

Sarris J; Byrne G J. (2010). A systematic review of insomnia and complementary medicine. *Sleep Medicine Reviews*. Apr;15(2):99-106. ISSN: 1087-0792

Schutte-Rodin S; Broch L; Buysse D; Dorsey C; Sateia M. (2008). Clinical guideline for the evaluation and management of chronic insomnia in adults. *J Clin Sleep Med*; 4(5):487-504.

Spielman AJ. (1986). Assessment of insomnia. *Clin Psychol Rev*. 6:11–25. ISSN: 0272-7358

Spielman A.J., Saskin P., Thorpy M.J. (1987). Treatment of chronic insomnia by restriction of time in bed. *Sleep*. 10: 45–56.

Szelenberger W., Skalski M. (1999). Epidemiologia zaburzeń snu w Polsce. Doniesienie wstępne. W: Nowicki Z., Szelenberger W. red. *Zaburzenia snu. Diagnostyka i leczenie, wybrane zagadnienia*. Biblioteka Psychiatrii Polskiej, Kraków; 57-63.

Szelenberger W. (2006). Standardy leczenia bezsenności Polskiego Towarzystwa Badań nad Snem. *Sen*, 2006, 6, supl. A:1-10.

Szelenberger w (ed.). (2007). *Bezsenność*. Via Medica, Gdańsk, 2007. ISBN 978-83-600072-61-5

Thase ME. (1999). Antidepressant treatment of the depressed patient with insomnia. *J Clin Psychiatry*. 60 (Suppl 17). 28–31. ISSN: 1555-2101

Walsh J, Roth T, Randazzo A, Erman M, Jamieson A, Scharf M, Schweitzer PK, Ware JC. (2000). Eight weeks of non-nightly use of zolpidem for primary insomnia. *Sleep*. 28:1087–96.

Winkelman JW, Buxton OM, Jensen JE, Benson KL, O'Connor SP, Wang W, Renshaw PF. (2008). Reduced Brain GABA in Primary Insomnia: Preliminary Data from 4T Proton Magnetic Resonance Spectroscopy (1H-MRS). *Sleep*, 31, 11:

World Health Organization (WHO). (1992). *The ICD-10 classification of mental and behavioral disorders: Clinical descriptions and diagnostic guidelines.* Geneva: world Health Organization.

Vgontzas AN, Tsigos C, Bixler EO, Stratakis CA, Zachman K, Kales A, Vela-Bueno A, Chrousos GP. (1998). Chronic insomnia and activity of the stress system: a preliminary study. *J Psychosom Res*, 45:21–31.

Yang CM, Spielman AJ, Huang, YS. (2005). Insomnia. *Current Treatment Options in Neurology*, 7:373–386

Part 3

Psychopharamcology of Insomnia

6

Treatment of Insomnia with Comorbid Mental Illness

Tracy L. Skaer
Professor of Pharmacotherapy, College of Pharmacy, Washington State University, USA

1. Introduction

Insomnia is the most prevalent sleep disorder; especially in the elderly.[1-3] It is diagnosed in women (55-60%) more often than men (40-45%).[4-6] It can occur acutely (as known as transient insomnia) or become a chronic disorder (occurring at least three or more times per week, usually one to six months in duration and with some degree of daytime dysfunction).[4] Epidemiological studies indicate that at least one symptom of insomnia occurs in approximately one-third of the adult population with about 10 to 15 percent of these cases suffering from chronic insomnia with daytime consequences lasting for months or for many, years.[4-10]

Chronic insomnia is frequently associated with depression and other psychiatric disorders including generalized anxiety disorder (GAD).[11-14] For some patients, insomnia symptoms may be a predictor for the onset of clinical depression.[12-16] Thus, given the potential for insomnia or its symptoms to reflect and/or trigger the onset of concomitant disease states, a thorough diagnostic examination is warranted in these patients.

Treatment guidelines for insomnia patients with comorbid mental illness are aimed at addressing the underlying psychiatric problem in order to improve sleep disturbances.[5,13] Successful treatment can only be achieved by a thorough understanding of the extent of the problem and the proper choice of interventions. A combination of lifestyle changes, psychiatric, complementary and alternative medicine, as well as pharmacotherapy are often employed to achieve a positive and lasting outcome.

2. Psychiatric comorbidities

The connection between insomnia and psychiatric comorbidities can be attributed to more than a simple cause and effect relationship. A bidirectional relationship has been identified in the literature.[17,18] Researchers have also determined that patients diagnosed with severe insomnia are 6 times more likely to have had a prior mental illness.[14] One study found that the odds of having at least one psychiatric diagnosis was 5.04 times greater in patients with severe insomnia as compared to those without insomnia and that increasing insomnia severity was associated with increased chronic medical and psychiatric illnesses. [19] Moreover, insomnia has been confirmed as a risk factor for future mental illness.[18]

3. Anxiety and depression

A prospective study conducted in Sweden showed that both anxiety and depression were associated with future insomnia and insomnia was associated with future anxiety and depression.[17] A baseline diagnosis of anxiety significantly predicted future insomnia, while an insomnia diagnosis at baseline significantly predicted future depression. A community-based retrospective study identified that chronic insomnia sufferers were about 10 times more likely to have clinically significant depression and about 17 times more likely to have clinically significant anxiety.[20] Chronic insomnia has been found to increase the risk of developing depression anywhere from 2 to 40 fold and those being treated for depression and have concomitant chronic insomnia are 2 to 4 times more likely to remain depressed if the insomnia remains untreated.[21-23]

4. Generalized anxiety disorder

The strong bidirectional association between chronic insomnia and anxiety disorders may indicate that they share an overlapping neurobiological abnormality with common symptoms and physiological markers (e.g. hyperarousal).[24] It is estimated that 70 to 90% of anxiety patients have insomnia as a complaint.[24,25] Two anxiety disorders, generalized anxiety disorder (GAD) and post traumatic stress disorder (PTSD) include sleep disturbance as part of the DSM-IV TR diagnostic criteria.

GAD has the highest comorbidity rate with insomnia; exceeding the comorbid rate of depression and insomnia.[11,25-27] Research estimates are as many as 50 to 70% of GAD sufferers have insomnia.[26] Additionally, sleep disturbances seem to worsen or trigger GAD-related symptoms of fatigue and irritability which are also hallmark consequences of insomnia.[26-27] Other overlapping symptomatology include excessive worry, significant daytime impairment, decreased sleep efficiency, increased nocturnal awakenings, and rapid eye movement (REM) sleep disturbances.[25,26]

5. Post traumatic stress disorder

PTSD patients commonly (70-90%) experience sleep disturbances.[26,27] These patients report sleep disturbance symptoms such as poor sleep quality, decreased total sleep time, nightmares, and hyerarousal.[26,27] Of important note, is that research has not demonstrated a bidirectional relationship between insomnia and PTSD given that an intervening trauma is necessary to establish a diagnosis of PTSD. Insomnia may predict the development of PTSD after trauma exposure however, and patients with more severe insomnia symptoms within a month of the trauma incident are at greater risk of developing PTSD within the following 12 month period.[26] Moreover, the severity of insomnia appears to be correlated with PTSD severity.[18]

6. Panic disorder

Empirical evidence exists to support the association between insomnia and panic disorder with about 67% of panic patients reporting difficulty falling asleep and 77% with difficulty maintaining sleep.[26,27] Approximately 44 to 77% of panic patients experience nocturnal panic attacks which have different pathology from those experienced during daylight hours.[27] A degree of hyperarousal may also be present.[25]

7. Comorbidity treatment stategies

Nearly 80% of patients diagnosed with major depressive disorder (MDD) have sleep disturbances with disturbed sleep and fatigue remaining after successful treatment of the mood disorder.[21,23,24,28,30] Lingering insomnia following treatment of depression is associated with increased risk of relapse (more than 50% of cases).[21,24,30] Therefore, insomnia is a significant independent predictor of future depression.[14,22-24,29] Clinical sequelae of insomnia such as negative affect, fatigue, anhedonia, poor concentration, and irritability are also symptoms found in depression. As mentioned earlier, a bidirectional relationship between depression and insomnia exists thereby emphasizing the importance of treating the insomnia independent of the comorbid condition.[24,28,31]

8. Treatment strategies

Several treatment strategies are utilized, often in various combinations, for the treatment of insomnia. These include psychological and behavioral therapy (PBT), pharmacotherapy, over-the-counter (OTC) medications, herbal and dietary supplements, complementary and alternative medicine (CAM), mind-body and lifestyle interventions (Table 1).

Lifestyle: sleep hygiene, weight control, low impact exercise, dietary (e.g. elimination of caffeine, nicotine, alcohol)
OTC medications: Not recommended by AASM and NIH
Herbal / Dietary supplements: melatonin (for changes in circadian rhythm, jet lag, shift work, or documented deficiency only); valerian (for acute treatment only)
PBT: stimulus control, coping skills, relaxation training (e.g. progressive muscle relaxation, guided imagery, abdominal breathing), CBT-I, multi-component therapy, sleep restriction, paradoxical intension, biofeedback, grief management
Mind and Body: yoga, meditation, mindfulness-based programs (MBSR, MBCT, MBT-I, MBRP), tai chi, acupuncture, acupressure
Pharmacological: SSRI or SNRI, augmentation with sedating antidepressant (low dose), BzRA (for acute treatment only), or benzodiazepine (minimal use: for acute or "as needed" treatment of anxiety symptoms only), prazosin

KEY: AASM = American Academy of Sleep Medicine; BzRA = benzodiazepine receptor agonist; CBT-I = cognitive behavioral therapy for insomnia; MBSR = mindfulness-based stress reduction; MBCT = mindfulness-based cognitive therapy; MBT-I = mindfulness based therapy for insomnia; MBRP = mindfulness-based relapse prevention; NIH = National Institutes of Health; OTC = over-the-counter; PBT Psychological and Behavioral Therapy; SNRI - serotonin norepinephrine receptor inhibitor; SSRI = selective serotonin reuptake inhibitor, TCA = tricyclic antidepressant

Table 1. Treatment Options for Insomnia with Co-Morbid Mental Illness

Unfortunately, clinicians are not routinely probing the level of sleep difficulties in their patients other than a simple identification (yes or no) of sleep disturbance.[32-38] Treatment seeking behavior for insomnia is based on disease severity, fatigue, daytime consequences and comorbidities.[32-33] A study of primary care patients with insomnia determined that the principal motivator for seeking treatment after controlling for insomnia severity was found to be the negative impact on daytime functioning.[32] A community based study identified that daytime fatigue and psychological distress were the main predictors of treatment seeking behavior.[5] Moreover, when patients seek treatment for their insomnia symptoms, health care providers (HCPs) are significantly more prone to prescribe pharmacotherapy than to refer patients for behavioral interventions.[34] Additionally, HCPs are more likely to diagnose one or more of the comorbidities as opposed to insomnia; there is a greater probability of obtaining reimbursement for these diagnoses by insurance carriers.[10,37,38] Thus, behavioral interventions which presume a diagnosis of insomnia remain underutilized.[37]

9. Sleep hygiene

A thorough evaluation of sleep hygiene is required at initial evaluation of all patients with sleeping difficulties. These simple and basic sleep practices offer a consistent routine to assist patients to return to a normal sleep schedule.[34,38-40] Adherence to good sleep hygiene practices is imperative in establishing a stable baseline to work from in order to improve sleeping difficulties. Sleep hygiene counseling includes the following:

- Follow a regular sleep pattern; go to bed and arise at about the same time each day.
- Eliminate daytime naps.
- Make the bedroom comfortable for sleeping by avoiding temperature extremes, noise and light.
- Make sure the bed is comfortable.
- Go to bed only when sleepy.
- Engage in relaxing activities before bedtime.
- Use the bed and bedroom only for sleep and sexual activities only.
- If unable to fall asleep, do not become anxious. Leave the bedroom and participate in relaxing activities for 20 to 30 minutes.
- If tense, practice relaxation exercises (e.g. deep breathing, meditation).
- If hungry, eat a light snack, but avoid eating meals or large snacks immediately before bedtime.
- Avoid using caffeine after noon.
- Avoid using alcohol or nicotine later in the evening.

Sleep hygiene is most effective when used in conjunction with other behavioral treatments. The overall goal is to decrease or eliminate sleep-reducing behaviors such as inconsistent sleep and wake cycle, daytime napping, clock monitoring, and exercising or consuming caffeine-containing beverages too close to bedtime.[39] One barrier to the success of sleep hygiene, is patient's perception that their compensatory behaviors of napping and drinking caffeinated beverages enable them to function during the day making them resistant to abandon these behaviors.[40] It is therefore recommended that HCPs be persistent in communicating their expectations on the importance of maintaining good sleep hygiene habits.

10. Over-the-counter remedies

Self-help remedies are a major source of treatments for many patients with insomnia. The most frequently used include over-the-counter (OTC) antihistamines (10-25%), herbal supplements, alcohol (10-25%), caffeinated beverages, or a diet high in carbohydrates and/or sugars throughout the day to combat fatigue.[5,41] None of these are suitable choices for the treatment of insomnia. Alcohol may reduce sleep-onset latency via its CNS depressive effects but it also disrupts sleep architecture causing disruption in REM and slow wave sleep.[42-44]

OTC antihistamines (e.g. diphenhydramine and doxylamine) are available for short term treatment of mild cases of insomnia only and should not be used for chronic insomnia. There is minimal evidence that these antihistamines are effective in improving sleep parameters but they may actually reduce sleep quality.[42,43] While these agents may help with mild cases of acute insomnia, they are not without potential serious adverse effects including daytime drowsiness, dizziness, fatigue, headaches, vomiting, and anticholinergic properties (e.g. blurred vision, urinary retention, confusion).[44-45] Moreover, the American Academy of Sleep Medicine (AASM) and the United States National Institutes of Health (NIH) both agree that there is insufficient evidence supporting the use of OTC antihistamines for the treatment of insomnia. This is of great concern as patients may experiment with various self-help remedies for a significant amount of time before consulting their HCP about their sleeping difficulties.

Many herbal and dietary supplements are marketed directly to the consumer as sleep aids however, consistent scientific evidence supporting their use is very limited.[42,44,46] Valerian and melatonin are the only supplements with sufficient research of adequate rigor evaluating their use in insomnia.[46] Unfortunately, recent meta-analyses of randomized clinical trials (RTCs) for valerian as monotherapy, or in combination with other herbal supplements, did not find significant improvement in sleep quality or sleep latency.[47,48]

Melatonin is a naturally occurring hormone that regulates sleep and circadian schedules. Research on melatonin's usefulness for insomnia is mixed. It has been primarily useful in decreasing sleep latency (e.g. jet lag, shift work-related insomnia) with no significant impact on sleep maintenance or total sleep time.[43-44] Additionally, melatonin has been associated with adverse effects such as residual fatigue, dizziness, headache, and irritability.[43,44] Therefore, it is not routinely recommended for treatment of chronic insomnia.

11. Psychological and behavioral therapy

PBT is considered first line treatment in chronic insomnia.[44] Unfortunately, it is under-utilized by practitioners even though there is significant evidence proving its effectiveness in chronic insomnia with or without comorbid illness.[30,36,44,49-51] Behavioral modification may actually be more useful for insomnia sufferers with comorbid illness as these patients are often burdened with a multitude of medications that enhance their risk for medication-related adverse effects, interactions, and/or dependency / addiction.[37]

It is hypothesized that physiological and cognitive hyperarousal contribute to the development and chronicity of insomnia.[44] Moreover, patients tend to develop problematic sleep hygiene practices such as remaining awake in bed for long periods of time which causes heightened anxiety and frustration about inability to sleep, increased efforts to sleep, wakefulness, negative expectations, and distorted attitudes about their insomnia and its consequences on their work/life. PBT is specifically targeted to address these perpetuating negative learned responses. The goal of PBT is to elicit a change in the patient's belief system, through education and awareness, which enhances the patient's sense of self-efficacy concerning their insomnia management.[44]

Relaxation training is often utilized with CBT-I and involves the use of progressive muscle relaxation, guided imagery, or abdominal breathing in order to lower somatic and cognitive arousal states that interfere with sleep. *Instructions:* PRM training involves the methodical tensing and relaxing of different muscle groups throughout the body. Techniques are widely available in written and audio formats.
Stimulus control is for the patient to establish a clear and positive association between the bed and sleep, as well as, creating a stable sleep-wake schedule. It is designed to eliminate the negative association between the bed and undesirable outcomes (e.g. wakefulness, frustration, worry) *Instructions:* Follow appropriate sleep hygiene
CBT-I is a combination of cognitive therapy with behavioral interventions (e.g., stimulus control, sleep restriction) with or without relaxation therapy. Cognitive therapy uses a psychotherapeutic method to reconstruct cognitive pathways with positive and appropriate concepts about sleep and its effects. CBT-I works to change the patient's overall beliefs and unrealistic expectations about sleep.
Multi-component therapy [without cognitive therapy] is employed by a majority of practitioners. It uses various combinations of behavioral interventions (e.g. stimulus control, relaxation, sleep restriction) and sleep hygiene education.
Sleep Restriction is used to improve sleep continuity by using sleep restriction to enhance sleep drive. The TIB to the TST is limited initially through the use of baseline sleep logs. As sleep drive increases and the window of sleep opportunity remains restricted with daytime napping prohibited, sleep becomes consolidated. As soon as sleep continuity significantly improves, TIB is slowly increased to provide adequate sleep time to feel rested during the day, while preserving the newly acquired sleep consolidation. *Instructions:* Patients should be cautioned that sleep restriction may create possible sleepiness and reduce cognition. Maintain sleep log and determine mean TST for a 1-2 week baseline; Set bedtime and wake-up times to approximate mean TST to achieve > 85% SE (TST/TIB x 100) over 1 week; the goal is for the TIB (not < 5 hrs) to be about the TST; Make weekly adjustments for SE > 85% to 90% over 1 week, TIB is increased by 15-20 minutes, for SE < 80%, TIB is decreased by 15-20 minutes; Repeat TIB adjustment every week until TST goal is achieved.
Paradoxical intention is used to eliminate anxiety over sleep performance. It is a targeted cognitive therapy which trains the patient to confront the fear of staying awake and its potential effects.
Biofeedback training is used to reduce somatic arousal. It trains the patient to control a selected physiologic variable through auditory or visual feedback.
Sleep hygiene teaches the patient healthy lifestyles that improve sleep. It is used in conjunction with stimulus control, relaxation training, sleep restriction, and/or CBT-I. *Instructions:* include, but are not limited to, keeping a regular sleep wake cycle, healthy dietary choices, regular daytime exercise program, maintaining a quiet sleep environment, avoidance of daytime napping, caffeine, nicotine, alcohol, other stimulants, excessive fluids, or stimulating activities before bedtime.

KEY: CBT-I = cognitive behavioral therapy for insomnia; PBT = psychological and behavioral therapy; SE = sleep efficiency; TIB = time in bed; TST = total sleep time.

Table 2. Common PBT for Chronic Insomnia

There are a number of different psychological and behavioral therapies available to address these aberrant behaviors (Table 2).[37,39,40,51-53] Standard therapies of stimulus control, relaxation training, and cognitive behavioral therapy for insomnia (CBT-I) with or without relaxation therapy are well supported in the scientific literature.[42,39,40,52,53] CBT-I is the most common form of PBT for chronic insomnia. CBT-I is individualized and combines several behavioral / multi-modal interventions. CBT-I usually includes stimulus control, sleep restriction, cognitive psychotherapy, light and dark exposure, sleep hygiene education, bedroom modification, relaxation training, and gradual tapering of hypnotic medications (when applicable).[44]

12. Complementary and alternative medicine

Pharmacotherapy and PBT interventions continue to be the mainstays of treatment for chronic insomnia patients with mental illness comorbidity. However, the use of complementary and alternative medicines (CAMs) has increased dramatically in the 21st century. CAMs (e.g. acupuncture, mindfulness-based stress reduction, yoga, meditation) are an integral part of the holistic medicine approach which aims to treat the "whole patient."[54] Patients are expected to play an active role in their health when receiving CAMs which appeals to many chronic sufferers who have experienced ineffective relief from conventional medicine practices. CAMs are increasingly becoming part of mainstream medicine as more research on their effectiveness is published.[54-60]

CAMs are more commonly used by those with psychiatric disorders especially patients with anxiety, depression and insomnia.[61-63] CAMs have shown to improve sleep in 4.5% of insomnia patients translating to 1.6 million U.S. citizens.[64] Herbal supplements or nutritional medicine, tai chi, and yoga are the most common CAMs utilized with 56% of patients reporting that CAMs were important in maintaining their health and 72% thought there was a significant improvement in their insomnia symptoms.[64]

Supportive evidence for acupuncture and acupressure in the treatment of insomnia is now available.[65-68] However, while acupuncture and acupressure may assist to improve sleep quality, the efficacy of these interventions was inconsistent between studies for many sleep parameters, including sleep onset latency, total sleep duration, and time to waking.[65-68] A recent study using electroacupucture for chronic insomnias demonstrated beneficial effects on sleep quality which, as the authors stated, may be associated with valuable repair of sleep architecture, reconstructing sleep continuity, prolonging slow wave sleep time and rapid eye movement (REM) sleep time.[57] Research using acupuncture and acupressure remains in progress and will hopefully demonstrate the full benefits as more rigorous studies are completed and published.

Mindfulness-based programs (utilizing meditation with or without yoga) have emerged as novel approaches to behavior modification, stress / anxiety reduction, pain management, and relapse prevention. Historically, meditation has been used to regulate physical and mental health and for spiritual development. Mindfulness meditation is an outgrowth from a Buddhist practice called *vipassana* ("to see a special way").[69] Mindfulness-based meditation is surfacing in Western cultures as a beneficial approach to patient healing for many chronic conditions (e.g. insomnia, chronic back pain, fibromyalgia, cancer, psoriasis)[70-73] This meditation technique fosters acute awareness of the present moment and the impermanent nature of things.[74] The patient is thereby able to cultivate the ability to respond to stimuli in a nonjudgmental way; allowing them to navigate their life in a manner that does not involve attachment to particular beliefs.[74] This form of self-compassion is the mechanism for reducing negative emotional reactions, enhancing resilience, and promoting self-healing.

There is a growing emphasis in applying mindfulness-based meditation in behavioral medicine. The first formal program, mindfulness-based stress reduction (MBSR) was created by Jon Kabat-Zinn over 2 decades ago and involves an 8-week program with an experiential component (formal mindfulness meditation) and group processing / support.[75] The MBSR program teaches patients how to make appropriate lifestyle changes by incorporating mindfulness techniques into their day-to-day life and encourages them to maintain a regular meditation practice. Several mindfulness-based programs have been designed from MBSR and adapted to meet the needs of specific populations. Mindfulness-based cognitive therapy (MBCT) is a program with assists in prevention and relapse of depression among individuals with recurrent major depressive disorders (MDD). MBCT could therefore be of benefit to those with insomnia and comorbid depressive illness.[76] Most recently, preliminary work on mindfulness-based therapy for insomnia (MBT-I) has been described as an effective treatment choice.[58-60] Additionally, there are also a mindfulness-based relapse prevention (MBRP) programs for depression, craving, as well as, alcohol and substance abuse.[77,78]

Low impact exercise, *Tai chi* and yoga are increasing in popularity as published research on mind-body interventions supports their use to improve sleep quality and reducing latency and insomnia severity.[79-81] Not all of these studies recruited chronic insomnia patients. Therefore, more yoga research is needed to validate its benefit for insomnia. Mainstream CAM studies including homoeopathy, massage, and aromatherapy are lacking at this time.

13. Pharmacotherapy

Currently there are no established treatment algorithms for insomnia with comorbid mental illness. While research has established the linkages between insomnia and psychiatric comorbidities, there is limited to no data to guide HCPs other than the reported recommendation to treat comorbidities (e.g. depression, GAD, PSTD, panic) concurrently, at recommended therapeutic doses, and in concert with PBT, sleep hygiene, and CAMs.[44]

Pharmacotherapy for comorbid insomnia can be effective, however, in improving targeted sleep parameters and improving symptoms of depression and anxiety disorders.[44,82-85] As mentioned earlier, treatment should address the insomnia and the comorbid mental illness simultaneously. Therapeutic choices include: benzodiazepine receptor agonists, selective serotonin reuptake inhibitors (SSRIs), serotonin and norepinephrine receptor antagonists (SNRIs), sedating antidepressants, anticonvulsants, and atypical antipsychotics.[44] Pharmacotherapy is not curative and therefore the best outcomes are realized when used in combination with other previous mentioned interventions (e.g. sleep hygiene, PBT, CAMs). Table 3 summarizes pharmacotherapy choices for insomnia with comorbid mental illness, as well as, various treatment considerations.

14. Sedative / hypnotics

While sedative hypnotic medications like eszopiclone, zolpidem, zaleplon, benzodiazepines (e.g. alprazolam, lorazepam, temazepam) have demonstrated efficacy for short-term treatment of insomnia, very little evidence exists to confirm their usefulness in chronic situations.[44]

Moreover, sedative hypnotics can produce residual sedation, memory and performance impairment, increased risk of falls and fractures, as well as, undesirable behaviors while sleeping (e.g. sleep walking, sleep driving, sleep talking).[44] Triazolam, for example, has been associated with rebound anxiety and is no longer considered a first line hypnotic.[44] Thus, these medications are best reserved for initial short-term therapy with the goal of little to no utilization once other interventions (e.g. antidepressant, PBT, sleep hygiene, CAMs) are successfully employed. Benzodiazepines, such as lorazepam, can be useful for immediate relief of breakthrough anxiety symptoms (e.g. panic attack) and prescribed on a limited "as needed" basis.[44] Buccal or sublingual administration of benzodiazepines provides rapid response and is very useful for these intense anxiety situations.

Medication	Therapeutic Considerations
BRAs: eszopiclone, zolpidem, zaleplon	For short term treatment of insomnia only; no evidence of efficacy in chronic situations.
BZDs: alprazolam, lorazepam, triazolam, temazepam	Best reserved for initial short term treatment of insomnia symptoms with the goal of little to no utilization once other interventions (e.g. SSRI, SNRI, PBT, sleep hygiene, CAMs) are successfully employed. May be used on a limited "as needed" basis for immediate relief of breakthrough anxiety symptoms (i.e. panic attack).
SSRIs: citalopram, escitalopram, fluoxetine, paroxetine, sertraline *SNRIs:* duloxetine, venlafaxine	"First line" for comorbid depression and/or anxiety disorders. Higher doses are often needed for anxiety disorders than for depression. Selection of medication is guided by treatment history, side effect profile, interactions with other medications, and expense. Citalopram and escitalopram have lowest propensity to interact with other medications.
Sedating Antidepressants: amitriptyline, doxepin, mirtazapine, nefazodone, trazodone, trimipramine	Use in low doses only; best used in combination as augmentation to SSRI or SNRI for treatment of persistent insomnia symptoms after an adequate trial of other interventions (e.g. SSRI, SNRI, PBT, sleep hygiene, CAMs). Limited evidence for trazodone and nefazodone as augmentation in PTSD. Do not use as monotherapy (weak efficacy).
Anticonvulsants: gabapentin, tiagavine Atypical Antipsychotics: olanzapine, quetiapine	Generally not recommended; limited evidence to support their use for chronic insomnia. Atypical antipsychotics show some promise in the treatment of anxiety disorders but their side effect profile (e.g, weight gain, metabolic syndrome) and noncompliance continue to limit their use.
Alpha Blocker: prazosin	For treatment of sleep disturbances (nightmares, disturbing dreams, insomnia) in PTSD. Recommended by the *AASM Best Practice Guide* for treatment of PTSD-related nightmares.

Key: AASM = American Academy of Sleep Medicine; BRA = benzodiazepine receptor agonist; BZD = benzodiazepine; CAM = complementary and alternative medicine; PBT = psychological and behavioral therapy; PTSD = post traumatic stress disorder; SNRI = serotonin and norepinephrine reuptake inhibitor; SSRI = selective serotonin reuptake inhibitor.

Table 3. Pharmacotherapy Choices for Insomnia and Comorbid Mental Illness

15. Antidepressants

Antidepressant (AD) medications, primarily SSRIs (e.g. citalopram, escitalopram, fluoxetine, paroxetine, sertraline) and SNRIs (e.g. duloxetine, venlafaxine), are first line for treatment of MDD, GAD, panic disorder, and PTSD.[86-88] These agents may or may not be effective in completely alleviating sleep disturbances. Therefore, low dose sedating antidepressants such as mirtazapine, doxepin, amitriptyline, or trimipramine, may be considered as augmentation when insomnia complaints continue even with adequate dosing of the SSRI or SNRI.[44] Moreover, low dose ADs are best used in combination with other antidepressant pharmacotherapy as their evidence for efficacy as monotherapy is rather weak.[89-94] Selection is primarily guided by treatment history, side effect profile, medications interactions and expense.[44] Elderly patients, for example, may not tolerate the anticholinergic side effects of trazadone, doxepin and amitriptyline. The weight gain associated with mirtazipine could be deleterious to diabetics, hyperlipidemics, or cardiovascular patients.

16. Anticonvulsants and atypical antipsychotics

Evidence to support the use of anticonvulsants (gabapentin, tiagabine) and atypical antipsychotics (quetiapine, olanzapine) for chronic insomnia is insufficient at this time.[44] Off-label use of these medications should not be recommended as they increase the potential for significant adverse effects (e.g. seizures with tigabine; weight gain and metabolic syndrome with quetiapine and olanzapine).[44] Additionally, atypical antipsychotics have been evaluated as monotherapy or augmentation in the treatment of anxiety disorders with or without comorbid MDD, schizophrenia, or bipolar disorder.[89] This recent critical evaluation of the available research confirmed that although atypical antipsychotics showed promising results in the treatment of anxiety disorders, their side effect profiles continue to limited their use.[89] Atypical antipsychotic side effects were found to be a source of non-compliance and resulted in premature discontinuation of treatment with higher dropout rates found in the majority of randomized clinical trials.[89]

17. Nefazodone, trazodone, and prazosin for PTSD

Nightmares and insomnia produce significant distress and daytime impairment in those with PTSD. There is limited evidence supporting the efficacy of nefazodone and trazodone augmentation in PTSD.[89] The *AASM Best Practice Guide* describes "low grade to sparse" data supporting trazadone use in this population and recommends against the use of nefazodone for the treatment of nightmares.[90] Fortunately, there is promising research using prazosin to treat sleep disturbances in PTSD.[85,91-93] Prazosin is the only medication to receive a grade of "recommended" by the *AASM Best Practice Guide* for the treatment of PTSD-related night mares.[90]

18. Conclusions and recommendations

Successful treatment of insomnia with comorbid mental illness is dictated by individualized treatment regimens where all appropriate options are considered. Treatment of both the insomnia and comorbid condition is important in achieving the best outcomes. Several treatment strategies in various combinations are often employed including sleep hygiene, PBT, CAMs, and pharmacotherapy. Behavioral modifications may actually be more useful for insomnia sufferers with comorbid illness as these patients are often burdened with a multitude of medications. Standard therapies of stimulus control, relaxation training, and CBT-I with or without insomnia are well supported in the literature. CAMs are commonly utilized in patients with anxiety, depression, and insomnia. Additionally, mindfulness-based programs (MBSR, MBCT, MBT-I, MBRP) are promising interventions and appear to be appropriate. Research on low-impact exercise (e.g. Tai chi and yoga) is currently emerging but certainly may be a beneficial lifestyle intervention in this population.

Selection of pharmacotherapy is based on a patient's treatment history, side effect profile, potential medication-related interactions, and expense. There are no established medication-related treatment algorithms for insomnia with comorbid mental illness. Sedative hypnotics have a limited role in these patients and are best reserved for initial short-term therapy with the goal of limited to no use after positive outcomes are demonstrated with other interventions. SSRIs and SNRIs are first line pharmacotherapy for MDD, GAD, panic disorder, and PTSD. SSRIs or SNRIs as monotherapy, however, may not be effective in completely alleviating the sleeping disturbances in these patients and augmentation therapy with sedating low-dose AD may be useful. The use of anticonvulsants and atypical antipsychotics in these patients is currently not well supported in the literature and the side effect profiles are problematic. Prazosin is now an AASM recommended medication for the treatment of sleep disorders associated with PTSD patients.

19. References

[1] Roth T. Insomnia: definition, prevalence, etiology, and consequences. *J Clin Sleep Med* 2007; 3(5 Suppl):S7-S10.

[2] Soldatos CR, Allaert FA, Ohta T, Dikeos DG. How do individuals sleep around the world? Results from a single day survey in ten countries. *Sleep Med* 2005: 6(1):5-13.

[3] Jaussent I, Bouyer J, Ancelin ML, et al. Insomnia and daytime sleepiness are risk factors for depressive symptoms in the elderly. *Sleep* 2011; 34(8):1103-10.

[4] Okayon MM, Gilleminault C. Epidemiology of sleep disorders. In: Chokroverty, S (Ed). *Sleep disorders medicine: basic science, technical considerations, and clinical aspects*, 4th Edition. Saunders, Philadelphia, PA, 2009, pp. 284-94.

[5] Morin CM, LeBlanc M, Daley M, et al. Epidemiology of insomnia: prevalence, self-help treatments, consultations, and determinants of help-seeking behaviors. *Sleep Med* 2006; 7(2):123-30.

[6] Doghramaji K. The epidemiology and diagnosis of insomnia. *Am J Manag Care* 2006; 12(8 Suppl.): S214-20.

[7] Thase ME. Correlates and consequences of chronic insomnia. *Gen Hosp Psychiatry* 2005; 27(2):100-12.

[8] LaBlanc M, Beaulieu-Bonneau S, Merette C, et al. Psychological and health related quality of life factors associated with insomnia in a population-based sample. *J Psychosom Res* 2007; 63(2):157-166.

[9] Ohayon MM. Difficulty in resuming or inability to resume sleep and the links to daytime impairment: definition, prevalence and comorbidity. *J Psychiatr Res* 2009; 43(10):934-40.

[10] Ozminkowski RJ, Wang S, Walsh JK. The direct and indirect costs of untreated insomnia in adults in the United States. *Sleep* 2007; 30(3):263-273.

[11] Ohayon MM, Reynolds CF. Epidemiological and clinical relevance of insomnia diagnosis algorithms, according to the DSM-IV and the international classification of sleep disorders (ICSD). *Sleep Med* 2009; 10(9):952-60.

[12] Johnson EO, Roth t, Breslau N. The association of insomnia with anxiety disorders and depression: exploration of the direction of risk. *J Psychiatr Res* 2006; 40(8):700-8.

[13] Riemann D. Insomnia and comorbid psychiatric disorders. *Sleep Med* 2007; 8(4 Suppl.):S15-S20.

[14] Ohayon MM, Roth T. Place of chronic insomnia in the course of depressive and anxiety disorders. *J Psychiatr Res* 2003; 37(1):9-15.

[15] Skaer TL, Robison LM, Sclar DA. Psychiatric comorbidity and pharmacological treatment patterns among patients presenting with insomnia: an assessment of office-based encounters in the USA in 1995 and 1996. *Clin Drug Investigation* 1999; 18(2):161-7.

[16] Skaer TL, Sclar DA, Robison LM. Complaint of insomnia in the United States 1995-1998: prevalence, psychiatric comorbidity, and pharmacologic treatment patterns. *Prim Care Psych*; 2001; 7(2):145-51.

[17] Jansson-Frojmark MJ, Lindbloom K. A bidirectional relationship between anxiety and depression, and insomnia? A prospective study in the general population. J *Psychosom Res* 2008; 64(4):443-49.

[18] Sateia MJ. Update on sleep and psychiatric disorders. *Chest* 2009; 135(5):1370-79.

[19] Sarsour K, Morin C, Foley K, Anupama K, Walsh JK. Association of insomnia severity and comorbid medical and psychiatric disorders in a health plan-based sample: insomnia severity and comorbidities. *Sleep Med* 2010; 11(1):69-74.

[20] Taylor D, Lichstein KL, Durrence HH, et al. Epidemiology of insomnia, depression, and anxiety. *Sleep* 2005; 28(11):1457-64.

[21] Manber R, Chambers AS, Insomnia and depression: a multifaceted interplay. *Curr Psychiatr Rep* 2009; 11(6):437-39

[22] Reinmann D, Voderholzer U. Primary insomnia: a risk factor for depression? *J Affect Dis* 2003; 76(1-3)255-59.

[23] Ebben, MR, Fine L. Insomnia: a risk for future psychiatric illness. In: Pandi-Paumal SR, Kramer M (eds), *Sleep and mental illness*. Cambridge University Press, Cambridge, UK. 2010, pp. 154-64.

[24] Ahmadi N, Saleh P, Shapiro CM. The association between sleep disorders and depression: implications for treatment. In: Pandi-Paumal SR, Kramer M (eds), *Sleep and mental illness*. Cambridge University Press, Cambridge, UK. 2010, pp. 154-64.

[25] Uhde TW, Cortese BM, Vedeniapin A. Anxiety and sleep problems: emerging concepts and theoretical treatment implications. *Curr Psychiatr Reprt* 2009; 11(4):269-76.

[26] Marcks A, Weisberg RB. Co-occurrence of insomnia and anxiety disorders: a review of the literature. *Am J Lifestyle Med* 2009; July/August: 300-9.

[27] Lee EK, Douglass AB. Sleep in psychiatric disorders: where are we now? *Can J Psych* 2010; 55(7):403-12.

[28] Van Mill JG, Hoogendijk MJG, Voelzangs N, et al. Insomnia and sleep duration in a large cohort of patients with major depressive disorder and anxiety disorders. *J Clin Psych* 2010; 71:239-46.

[29] Neckelmann D, Mykletun A, Dahl AA. Chronic insomnia as a risk factor for developing anxiety and depression. *Sleep* 2007; 30(7):873-79.

[30] Dombrovski AY, Cyranowski JM, Mulsant BH, et al. Which symptoms predict recurrence of depression in women treated with maintenance interpersonal psychotherapy? *Depress Anxiety* 2008; 25(12):1060-66.

[31] Neubauer DN. Current and new thinking in the management of comorbid insomnia. *Am J Manag Care* 2009; 15(suppl):S24-S32.

[32] Aikens JE, Rouse ME. Help-seeking for insomnia among adult patients in primary care. *J Am Board Fam Pract* 2005; 18(4):257-261.

[33] Bartless D, Marshall NS, Williams A, Grunstein RR. Predictors of primary medical care consultations for sleep disorders. *Sleep Med* 2008; 9(8):857-864.

[34] Hamblin JE. Insomnia: an ignored health problem *Primary Care Clin in Office Pract* 2007; 34(3):569-74.

[35] Ohayon MM. Nocturnal awakenings and comorbid disorders in the American general population. *J Psych Res* 2009; 43(1):48-54.

[36] Thase EM. Correlates and consequences of chronic insomnia. *Gen Hosp Psych* 2005; 27:100-12.

[37] Rybarczyk B, Lund HG, Mack I, Stepanski E. Comorbid insomnia. *Sleep Med Med Clinics* 2009; 4:571-82.

[38] Sorscher AJ. How is your sleep: a neglected topic for health care screening? *J Am Board Fam Med* 2008; 21(2):141-148.

[39] Ebben MR, Spielman AL. Non-pharmacological treatments for insomnia. *J Behave Med* 2009; 32(3):244-254.

[40] Yang CM, Spielman AJ, Glovinsky P. Nonpharmacologic strategies in the management of insomnia. *Psych Clinic N Amer* 2006; 29(4):895-919.

[41] Morin, CM. Beaulieu-Bonneau S, LeBlanc M, Savard J. Self-help treatment for insomnia: a randomized controlled trial. *Sleep* 2005; 28(10):1319-1327.

[42] Meoli AL, Rosen C, Kristo D, et al. Oral nonprescription treatment for insomnia: an evaluation of products with limited evidence. *J Clin Sleep Med* 2005; 1(2):173-87.

[43] Ramakrishnan K, Scheid DC. Treatment options for insomnia. *Am Fam Physician* 2007; 76(4):517-26.

[44] Schutte-Rodin S, Broch L, Buysse D, et al. Clinical guideline for the evaluation and management of chronic insomnia in adults. *J Clin Sleep Med* 2008; 4(5):487-504.

[45] Bain KT. Management of chronic insomnia in elderly persons. *Am J Geriatr Pharmacother* 2006; 4(2):168-92.

[46] Sarris J, Panossian A, Scheweiterzer I, et al. Herbal medicine for depression, anxiety and insomnia: a review of psychopharmacology and clinical evidence. *Eur Neuoropsychopharm* 2011; in press.

[47] Bent S, Padula A, Moore D, et al. Valerian for sleep: a systematic review and meta-analysis. *Am J Med* 2006; 119(12):1005-1012

[48] Fernandex-San-Martin MI, Masa-Font R, Palacios-Soler L, et al. Effectiveness of valerian on insomnia: a meta-analysis of randomized placebo-controlled trials. *Sleep Med* 2010; 11(6):505-11.

[49] Morin CM, Bootzin RR, Buysse DJ, et al. Psychological and behavioral treatment of insomnia: update of recent evidence. *Sleep* 2006; 29(11):1398-1414.

[50] Morgenthaler T, Kramer M, Alessi C, et al. Practice parameters for the psychological and behavioral treatment of insomnia: an update. An American Academy of Sleep Medicine Report. *Sleep* 2006; 29(11):1415-19.

[51] Stepanski EJ, Rybarczyk B. Emerging research on the treatment and etiology of secondary or comorbid insomnia. *Sleep Med Rev* 2009; 10(1):7-18.
[52] Siebern AT, Manber R. Insomnia and its effective non-pharmacologic treatment. *Med Clinical N Amer* 2010; 94(3):581-91.
[53] Taylor DJ, Roane BM. Treatment of insomnia in adults and children: a practice-friendly review of research. *J Clin Psych* 2010; 66(11):1137-1147.
[54] Sarris J, Byrne GJ. A systematic review of insomnia and complementary medicine. *Sleep Med Rev* 2011; 15(2):99-106.
[55] Kozasa EH, Hachul H, Monson C, et al. Mind-body interventions for the treatment of insomnia: a review. *Rev Bras Psiquiatr* 2010; 32(4):37-43.
[56] Hughes CM, McCullough CA, Bradbury I, et al. Acupuncture and reflexology for insomnia: a feasibility study. *Acupunct Med* 2009; 27(4):163-68.
[57] Ruan JW, Wang CH, Liao XX et al. Electroacupuncture treatment of chronic insomniacs. *Chin Med J* 2009; 122(23):2869-2873.
[58] Ong JC, Shapiro SL, Manber R. Combining mindfulness meditation with cognitive-behavior therapy for insomnia: A treatment-development study. *Behav Therap* 2008; 39(2):171-82.
[59] Ong JC, Sholtes D. A mindfulness-based approach to the treatment of insomnia. *J Clin Psych* 2010; 66(11):1175-84.
[60] Ong JC, Shapiro SL, Manber R. Mindfulness meditation and cognitive behavioral therapy for insomnia: a naturalistic 12-month follow-up. *Explore* 2009; 5(1):30-6.
[61] Kessler RC, Soukup J, Davis RB, et al. The use of complementary and alternative therapies to treat anxiety and depression in the United States. *Am J Psychiatry* 2001; 158(2):289-94.
[62] Elkins G, Rajab MH, Marcus J. Complementary and alternative medicine use by psychiatric inpatients. *Psychol Rep* 2005; 96(1):163-6.
[63] Sanchez-Ortuno M, Belanger L, Ivers H, et al. The use of natural products for sleep: a common practice? *Sleep Med* 2009; 10(9):982-7.
[64] Pearson NJ, Johnson LL, Nahin RL. Insomnia, trouble sleeping and complementary and alternative medicine: analysis of the 2002 national health interview survey data. *Arch Intern Med* 2006; 166(16):1775-82.
[65] Huang W, Kutner N, Bliwise DL. A systematic review of the effects of acupuncture in treating insomnia. *Sleep Med Rev* 2009; 10(9):982-7
[66] Yeung WF, Chung KF, Leung YK, et al. Traditional needle acupuncture treatment for insomnia: a systematic review of randomized controlled trials. *Sleep Med* 2009; 10(7):694-704.
[67] Cheuk DKL, Yeung WF, Chung KF, Wong V. Acupuncture for insomnia. Cochrane Database of *Syst Rev* 2007; July 18(3): CD005472.
[68] Chen HY, Shi Y, Ng CS, et al. Auricular acupuncture treatment for insomnia: a systemic review. *J Altern Complement Med* 2007; 13(6):669-76.
[69] Chavan DV. Vipassana: The Buddha's tool to probe mind and body. *Prog Brain Res* 2008; 168:247-53.
[70] Morone NE, Greco CM, Weiner DK. Mindfulness meditation for the treatment of chronic low back pain in older adults: A randomized controlled pilot study. *Pain* 2008; 134(3):310-19.

[71] Grossman P, Tiefenthaler-Gilmer U, Raysz A, Kesper U. Mindfulness training as an intervention for fibromyalgia: Evidence of post-intervention and 3-year follow-up benefits in well-being. *Psychother Psychosom* 2007; 76(4):226-233.
[72] Carlson L, Garland S. Impact of mindfulness-based stress reduction (MBSR) on sleep, mood, stress and fatigue symptoms in cancer outpatients. *Int J Behav Med* 2005; 12(4):278-85.
[73] Kabat-Zinn J, Wheeler E, Light T, et al. Influence of a mindfulness meditation-based stress reduction intervention on rates of skin clearing in patients with moderate to severe psoriasis undergoing phototherapy (UVB) and photochemotherapy (PUVA). *Psychosom Med* 1998; 60(5):625-32.
[74] Ludwig D, Kabat-Zinn J. Mindfulness in medicine. *JAMA* 2008; 300(11):1350-52.
[75] Kabat-Zinn J. *Full catastrophic living: Using the wisdom of your body and mind to face stress, pain, and illness.* Batam Dell: a division of Random House, Inc. New York, NY. 1990.
[76] Segal ZV, Williams JMG, Teasdale JD. Metacognitive awareness and prevention of relapse in depression: Empirical evidence. *J Consult Clin Psychol* 2002; 70(2):275-87.
[77] Witkiewitz K, Marlatt GA, Walker D. Mindfulness based relapse prevention for alcohol and substance use disorders. *J Cogn Psychother* 2005; 19(2):211-28.
[78] Witkiewitz K, Bowen S. Depression, craving, and substance abuse following a randomized trial of mindfulness-based relapse prevention. *J Consul Clin Psychol* 2010; 78(3):362-74.
[79] Montgomery P, Dennis J. Physical exercise for sleep problems in adults aged 60+. *Cochrane Database Syst Rev* 2002:4:CD003404.
[80] Li F, Fisher KJ, Harmer P, et al. Tai chi and self-rated quality of sleep and daytime sleepiness in order adults: A randomized controlled trial. *J Am Geriatr Soc* 2004; 52(6):892-900.
[81] Manjunath NK, Telles S. Influence of Yoga and Ayurveda on self-rated sleep in geriatric population. *Indian J Med Res* 2005; 121(5):683-90.
[82] Roth T. Comorbid insomnia: current directions and future challenges. *Am J Manag Care* 2009; 15 (suppl):S6-S13.
[83] Krystal Ad. A compendium of placebo-controlled trials of the risks / benefits of pharmacological treatments for insomnia: The empiric basis of U.S. Clinical practice. *Sleep Med Rev* 2009; 13(4):265-74.
[84] Steckler T, Risbrough V. Pharmacological treatment of PTSD: Established and new approaches. *Neuropharmacol* 2011, in press.
[85] Nappi CM, Drummond SPA, Hall JMH. Treating nightmares and insomnia in posttraumatic stress disorder: A review of current evidence. *Neuropharmacol* 2011: in press.
[86] Davidson JR, Zhang W, Connor KM, et al. A psychopharmacological treatment algorithm for generalized anxiety disorder (GAD). *J Psychopharmacol* 2010;24(1):3-26.
[87] Baldwin DS, Anderson IM, Nutt DJ, et al. Evidence-based guidelines for the pharmacological treatment of anxiety disorders: Recommendations from the British Society for Psychopharmacology. *J Psychopharmacol* 2005; 19(6):567-596.
[88] American Psychiatric Association. Practice Guideline for the treatment of patients with panic disorders, second edition. 2009 http://www.psychiatryonline.com/pracGuide/pracGuideTopic_9.aspx. Website access: September 15, 2011.

[89] Neylan TC, Lenoci M, Maglione ML, et al. The effect of nafazodone on subjective and objective sleep quality in posttraumatic stress disorder. *J Clin Psychiatry* 2003; 64(4):445-50.
[90] Aurora RN, Zak RS, Auerbach SH, et al. Best practice guide for the treatment of nightmare disorder in adults. *J Clin Sleep Med* 2010; 6(4):389-401.
[91] Berger W, Mendlowicz MV, Marques-Portella C, et al. Pharmacologic alternatives to antidepressants in posttraumatic stress disorder: A systematic review. *Prog Neuropsychopharm Biol Psychiatry* 2009; 33(2):169-80.
[92] Maher MJ, Rego SA, Asnis GM. Sleep disturbances in patients with post-traumatic stress disorder: epidemiology, impact and approaches to management. *CNS Drugs* 2006; 20(7):567-90.
[93] Miller LJ. Prazosin for the treatment of posttraumatic stress disorder sleep disturbances. *Pharmacother* 2008; 28(5):656-66.

7

Structural Relationship Study of Octanol-Water Partitioning Coefficients and Total Biodegradation of Barbiturate Medicines by Randić Descriptor

Avat (Arman) Taherpour[1*], Zhiva Taherpour[2] and Omid Taherpour[3]
[1]*Chemistry Department, Graduate School, Islamic Azad University, Arak Branch,*
[2]*Cardiology Department, Golestan Hospital, Ahwaz,*
[3]*Dentistry Faculty, Centro Escolar University,*
[1,2]*Iran*
[3]*Philippines*

1. Introduction

Insomnia is most often defined by an individual's report of sleeping difficulties.[1] One definition of insomnia is difficulties in initiating and maintaining sleep, or non-restorative sleep, associated with impairments of daytime functioning or marked distress for more than 1 month."[1,2] insomnia is most often thought of as both a sign[1,3] and a symptom[1,4] that can accompany several sleep, medical, and psychiatric disorders, characterized by persistent difficulty falling asleep and staying asleep or sleep with bad quality. Specialists in sleep medicine have been attempted to diagnose many different sleep disorders. Patients with various disorders including delayed sleep phase syndrome are often misdiagnosed as primary insomnia. When a person has trouble for getting to sleep but has a normal sleep pattern once asleep, circadian rhythm disorder has almost the same cause. In many cases, insomnia is co-morbid with another disease, side-effects of medications, or a psychological problem. Approximately half of all causes of insomnia are related to psychiatric disorders.[1-4] It is possible that insomnia represents a significant risk for the development of a subsequent psychiatric disorder."[1] Sleep-onset insomnia is difficulty falling asleep at the beginning of the night, often a symptom of anxiety disorders or the delayed sleep phase disorder.

There are two types of insomnia: primary insomnia and secondary insomnia. Primary insomnia means that a person having sleep problems that are not directly associated with any other health condition or problem. Secondary insomnia means that a person having sleep problems because of something else, such as a health condition (like asthma, depression, arthritis, cancer, or heartburn); pain; medication they are taking; or a substance they are using (like alcohol and other compounds).[5-9]

* Corresponding Author

Pharmacological treatments have been used mainly to reduce symptoms in acute insomnia; their role in the management of chronic insomnia remains unclear.[1-4]It is important to identify or rule out medical and psychological causes before deciding on the treatment for insomnia.[1,10] Attention to sleep hygiene is an important first line treatment strategy and should be tried before any pharmacological approach is considered.[1,11]

2. Barbiturates

Barbiturates are drugs that act as central nervous system depressants. By virtue of this, they produce a wide spectrum of effects, from mild sedation to total anesthesia. Barbiturates are also effective as anxiolytics, hypnotics, and anticonvulsants.[12] Barbiturates are still widely used in surgical anesthesia, especially to induce anesthesia. These compounds are derivatives of barbituric acid. Barbituric acid was first synthesized in 1864, by Adolf von Baeyer. The synthesis was done by condensing urea (an animal waste product) with diethyl malonate.[12,13] Barbiturates were first introduced for medical use in the early 1900s. More than 2,500 barbiturates have been synthesized, and at the height of their popularity, about 50 were marketed for human use. Barbiturates produce a wide spectrum of central nervous system depression, from mild sedation to coma, and have been used as sedatives, hypnotics, anesthetics, and anticonvulsants. The primary differences among many of these products are how fast they produce an effect and how long those effects last. Barbiturates are classified as ultra-short, short, intermediate, and long-acting. The Ultra-short barbiturates such as thiopental (Pentothal) produce unconsciousness within about a minute of intravenous (IV) injection. These drugs may be used to induce general anesthesia. Volatile anesthetics are then used to maintain general anesthesia until the end of the operation. Because thiopental and other ultrashort-acting barbiturates are typically used in hospital settings, they are not very likely to be abused, noted the DEA.[12] Barbiturate abusers prefer the short-acting and intermediate-acting barbiturates. After oral administration, the onset of action is from 15 to 40 minutes, and the effects last up to six hours. These drugs are primarily used for insomnia and preoperative sedation. Veterinarians use pentobarbital for anesthesia and euthanasia. Long-acting barbiturates include phenobarbital (Luminal) and mephobarbital (Mebaral). Effects of these drugs are realized in about one hour and last for about 12 hours, and are used primarily for daytime sedation and the treatment of seizure disorders. Barbiturates contain a "balance" of hydrophilic (2,4,6-pyrimidinetrione ring structure) and lipophilic (5,5′-substituents) functionality. The overall hydrophilic (polar) or lipophilic (non-polar) character of the barbiturates is a function of: the hydrophilicity of the pyrimidinetrione ring which is a function of the number of N-substituents and the pKa of the acidic proton(s), and the overall size and structure of the two substituents at the 5-position. (See Fig.-1).[14-19]

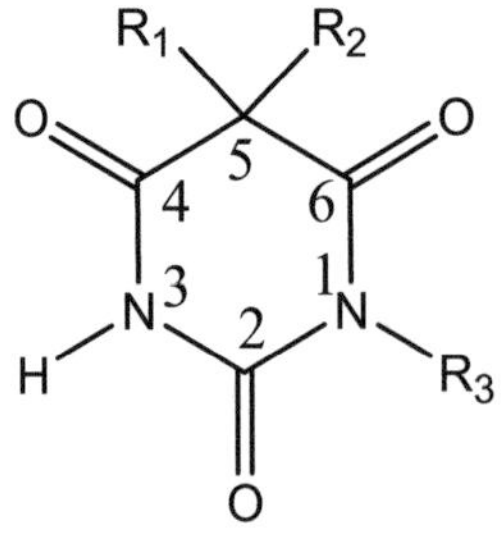

Common Barbiturates structure

2.1 Mechanism of barbiturates action

The principal mechanism of action of barbiturates is believed to be their affinity for the $GABA_A$ receptor (acts on GABA (Gamma-aminobutyric acid; $H_2N(CH_2)_3COOH$):benzodiazepine (BDZ) receptor Cl^- channel complex). The GABA receptors are a class of receptors that respond to the neurotransmitter gamma-aminobutyric acid (GABA), the chief inhibitory neurotransmitter in the vertebrate central nervous system.[14,15] There are two classes of GABA receptors: $GABA_A$ and $GABA_B$. $GABA_A$ receptors are ligand-gated ion channels (also known as ionotropic receptors), whereas $GABA_B$ receptors are G protein-coupled receptors (also known as metabotropic receptors). Barbiturates bind to the $GABA_A$ receptor at the alpha subunit, which are binding sites distinct from GABA itself and also distinct from the benzodiazepine binding site.[20,21] Like benzodiazepines, barbiturates have similar effect of GABA at this receptor. In addition to this GABA-ergic effect, barbiturates also block the AMPA (α-amino-3-hydroxy-5-methyl-4-isoxazolepropionic acid) receptor, a subtype of glutamate receptor.[20,21] The AMPA receptor (AMPAR, or quisqualate receptor) is a non ionotropic trans-membrane receptor types for glutamate that mediates fast synaptic transmission in the central nervous system (CNS). Its name is derived from its ability to be activated by the artificial glutamate analog AMPA.[21] Barbiturates produce their pharmacological effects by increasing the duration of chloride ion channel opening at the $GABA_A$ receptor, increases the efficacy of GABA, whereas benzodiazepines increase the frequency of the chloride ion channel opening at the $GABA_A$ receptor to increase the potency of GABA. The direct gating or opening of the chloride ion channel is the reason for the increased toxicity of barbiturates compared to benzodiazepines in overdose.[20-23]

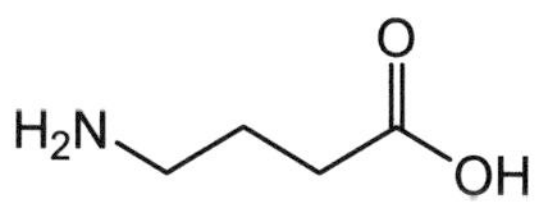

GABA

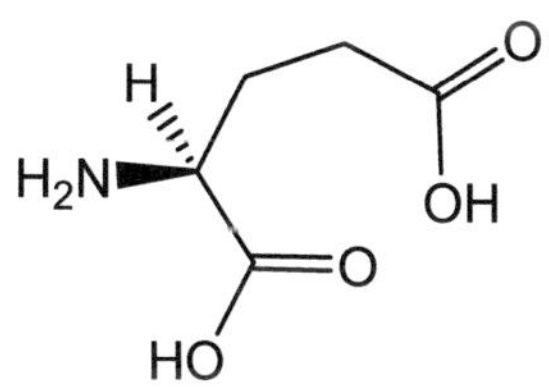

Glutamic Acid

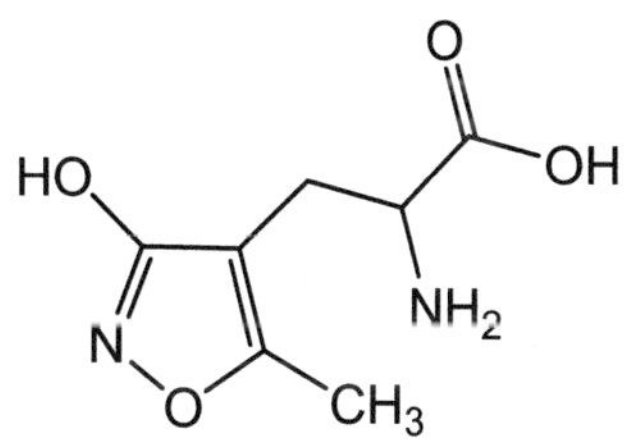

AMPA

Barbiturates are relatively non-selective compounds that bind to an entire super-family of ligand-gated ion channels, of which the $GABA_A$ receptor channel is only one of several representatives. While $GABA_A$ receptor currents are increased by barbiturates (and other general anaesthetic compounds), ligand-gated ion channels that are predominantly permeable for cationic ions are blocked by these compounds.[12,24] The findings implicate (non-GABA-ergic) ligand-gated ion channels in mediating some of the (side) effects of barbiturates.[12,25]

In 1988, the synthesis and binding study of an artificial receptor binding barbiturates by 6 complementary hydrogen bonds was published by Chang and Hamilton.[26] According to this study, different kinds of receptors were designed, as well as different barbiturates and cyanurates, not for their efficiencies as drugs but for applications in supramolecular chemistry, in the conception of materials and molecular devices.[12,26] The actions of the barbiturates are described in more detail in the Pharmacology Notes. General properties of these compounds relatively concern to low *"lipophilicity"* and low plasma protein binding.[14-20]

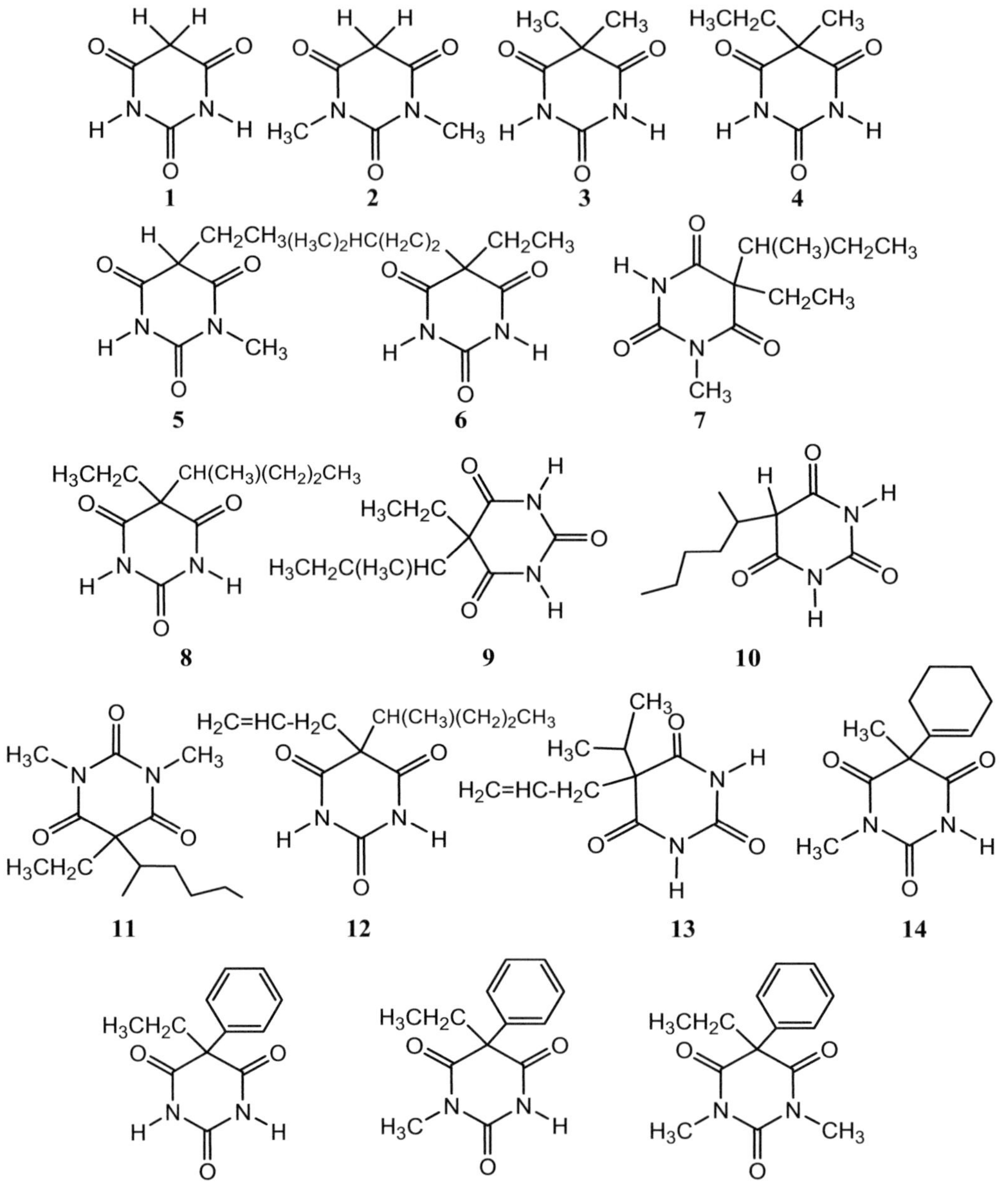

Fig. 1. The Barbiturates **1-17** structures.

3. Octanol-water partition coefficient and biodegradation of barbiturates

The octanol-water partition coefficient (K_{ow}) is a measure of the equilibrium concentration of a compound between octanol and water that indicates the potential for partitioning in to soil organic matter (i.e., a high K_{ow} indicates a compound which will preferentially partition into soil organic matter rather than water). This coefficient is inversely related to the solubility of a compound in water. The $logK_{ow}$ is used in models to estimate plant and soil invertebrate bioaccumulation factors. The $logK_{ow}$ is commonly used in QSAR studies and drug design, since this property is related to drug absorption, bioavailability, metabolism, and toxicity. This parameter is also used in many environmental studies to help determine the environmental fate of chemicals.[27,28] It has quite a lot of use in medicine and medicinal chemistry. Biodegradation (TB_d in mol/h)) is another useful and important factors in chemical and biochemical studies.[28]

It needs to use the effective and useful mathematical methods for making good concern between several data of chemical properties, medicinal chemistry and biological activity of chemicals.

Graph theory is an attractive field for the exploration of proof techniques in *Discrete Mathematics* and its results have applications in many areas of sciences. A graph is a topological concept rather than a geometrical concept of fixed geometry, and hence Euclidean metric lengths, angles and three-dimensional spatial configurations have no meaning.

Chemists employ various types of names and formulas when they wish to communicate information about chemicals and their structures. For the most part names and formulas have no direct, immediate or explicit mathematical meaning. Graph theory provides many different methods of characterizing chemical structures numerically.

It has been found to be a useful tool in *QSAR* (Quantitative Structure Activity Relationship) and *QSPR* (Quantitative Structure Property Relationship).[29-34] Numerous studies have been made relating to the above mentioned fields by using what are called topological indices (TI).[34,35]

In this study, will be considered the relationship of *Randić* index, for molecular description of structure-property relationship studies for the logarithm of calculated Octanol-Water partitioning coefficients and total biodegradation ($logK_{ow}$ and TB_d (mol/h), respectively) in Barbiturate compounds **(1-17)**.

4. Mathematical operations

The branching index that was introduced by *Randić* is defined as the sum of certain bond contributions calculated from the degree of the bonds suppressed molecular graphs. These bond contributions, named C_{ij} are calculated as:

$$C_{ij} = (\delta_i \, \delta_j)^{-0.5} \tag{1}$$

Where δ_i is the degree of the vertex representing atom "*i*", i.e., the number of bonds incident to this atom. Accordingly, the *Randić* index is defined as: [29,35-38]

$$\chi = \Sigma C_{ij} = \Sigma(\delta_i \, \delta_j)^{-0.5} \tag{2}$$

Where the summation is carried out over all the bonds of **1-17**.

The inverse squared–root of the vertex degree is identified here as a measure of the relative accessible perimeter of an atom from the outside. These perimeters, which have length units, are proposed to be measured in a new unit called the *Randić* index (χ). On this basis, the bond contributions to the *Randić* index are relative areas of bond accessibility from the environment.

All graphing operations were performed using the *Microsoft Office Excel-2003* program.The data of Octanol-Water partitioning coefficients and total biodegradation ($logK_{ow}$ and TB_d, respectively) were calculated by EPI-suit v3.12 package [39].

5. Results and discussion

It was accepted that the organic compounds toxicity properties can be introduced by utilizing the $logK_{ow}$.[40] The quantitative structural activities and properties relationship results hold true for quite a lot of organic compounds, the most commonly used for test organism, follows this standard pattern. [41] Biodegradation is usually quantified by incubating a chemical compound in presence of a degrader, and measuring some factors like oxygen or production of CO_2. The biodegradation QSAR studies demonstrate that microbial biosensors are a viable alternative means of reporting on potential biotransformation. However, a few chemicals are tested and large data sets for different chemicals need for QSAR modeling [42]. This study shows the structural relationship between *Randić* index (χ), $logK_{ow}$ and total biodegradation (TB_d) for barbiturates **(1-17)**. The values of the relative structural coefficients of the barbiturates structures **(1-17)**, *Randić* index (χ) to logarithm of Octanol-Water partitioning coefficients ($logK_{ow}$) and calculated total biodegradation (TB_d) in mol/h, data were shown in Table-1. The χ values of **1-17** increase with the increasing the number of branches in the appropriate structures. The *Randić* index (χ) for barbituric acid **(1)** in respect with the branches of the structure is equal to 2.1216. See equations 1 and 2 and the appropriate data extended in Table-1 for other members of these group.

$$\chi = 6[(2\times4)^{-0.5}]= 2.1216$$

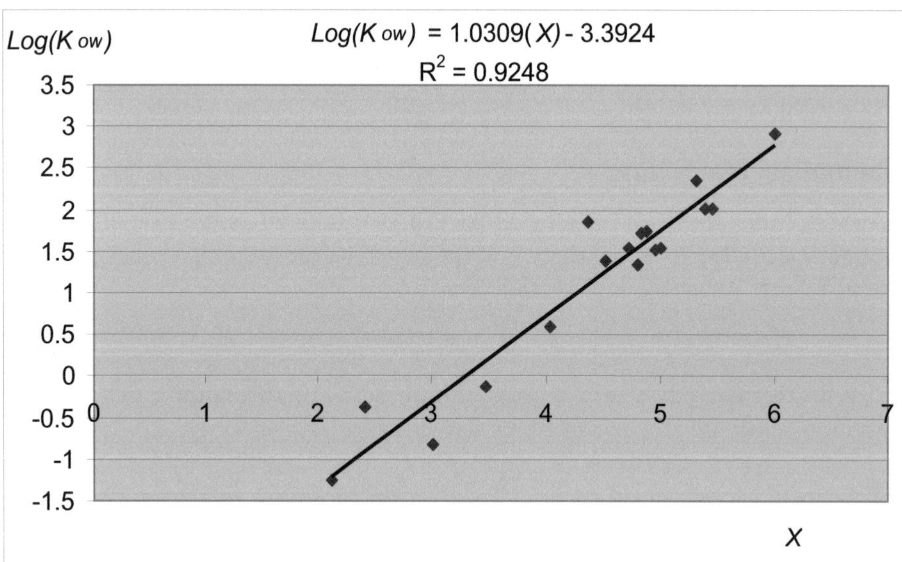

Fig. 2. The linear relationship between the values of log(K_{ow}) versus the Randic Indices (χ) for Barbiturates **(1-17)**.

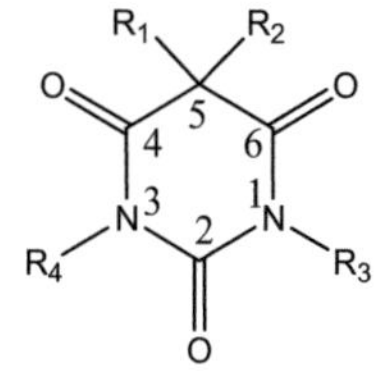

No.	R_1	R_2	R_3	R_4	Randic Indices (χ)	Log K_{ow}	$TB_d \times 10^{-5}$ (mol/h)
1	H	H	H	H	2.1216	-1.2488	7.2
2	H	H	CH_3	CH_3	3.0166	-0.8264	5.9
3	CH_3	CH_3	H	H	2.4144	-0.3777	5.9
4	H	H	CH_3	C_2H_5	3.4751	-0.1289	5.4
5	CH_3	H	C_2H_5	H	4.0358	0.6045	5.0
6	$(CH_2)_2CH(CH_3)_2$	C_2H_5	H	H	5.3911	2.0043	4.2
7	$CH(CH_3)CH_2CH_3$	C_2H_5	CH_3	H	4.8266	1.7244	4.1
8	$CH(CH_3)(CH_2)_2CH_3$	C_2H_5	H	H	5.4564	2.0043	4.3
9	$CH(CH_3)CH_2CH_3$	C_2H_5	H	H	4.9564	1.5132	4.4
10	$CH(CH_3)(CH_2)_3CH_3$	H	H	H	4.7188	1.5508	4.4
11	$CH(CH_3)(CH_2)_3CH_3$	C_2H_5	CH_3	CH_3	5.9978	2.9178	4.4
12	CH_2-CH=CH2	$CH(CH_3)(CH_2)_2CH_3$	H	H	5.3152	2.3590	4.0
13	CH_2-CH=CH2	$CH(CH_3)_2$	H	H	4.5277	1.3768	4.4
14	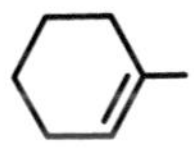	CH_3	CH_3	H	4.3593	1.8548	3.8
15	C_6H_5-	C_2H_5	H	H	4.8025	1.3301	4.0
15	C_6H_5-	C_2H_5	CH_3	H	5.0059	1.5413	3.8
17	C_6H_5-	C_2H_5	CH_3	CH_3	4.8761	1.7525	3.6

Table 1. The values of the relative structural coefficients of Barbiturates structures **(1-17)**.

In Fig.-2 to Fig.-4 were shown two dimensional diagrams of the relationship between the values of *Randić* index, $logK_{ow}$ and TB_d.

The figure 2 shows a good linear relationship between the values of $\log(K_{ow})$ versus the Randic Indices (χ) for barbiturates **(1-17)**. The Eq.-3 is relevant to Fig.-2, and as could see by this equation can extend the linear behavior of the calculated $logK_{ow}$ and χ for these compounds. The R-squared value (R^2) for this graph is equal to 0.9248.

$$log(K_{ow}) = 1.0309(\chi) - 3.3924 \qquad (3)$$

By this way, equation 3 afford a good approximation for calculation of logarithm value of Octanol-Water partitioning coefficient ($log\ K_{ow}$) by the use of *Randić* index (χ) and directly for the barbiturates. The large values results for solving the first order Eq.-3 are acceptable. For achieving to $logK_{ow}$ can use directly from Eq.-3, in accordance with the structural "χ" values for these compounds.

The Fig.-3 shows a curve for relationship between the values of calculated total biodegradation (TB_d) versus the Randic Indices (χ) for **1-17**. The Eq.-4 is relevant to Fig.-4, and can see the non linear behavior of the calculated total biodegradation (TB_d) and χ for barbiturates **(1-17)**. The equation has three-order structure. The R-squared value (R^2) for this graph shows 0.8916.

$$TB_d = 0.0825(\chi)^3 - 0.7268(\chi)^2 + 0.901(\chi) + 7.4083 \quad (4)$$

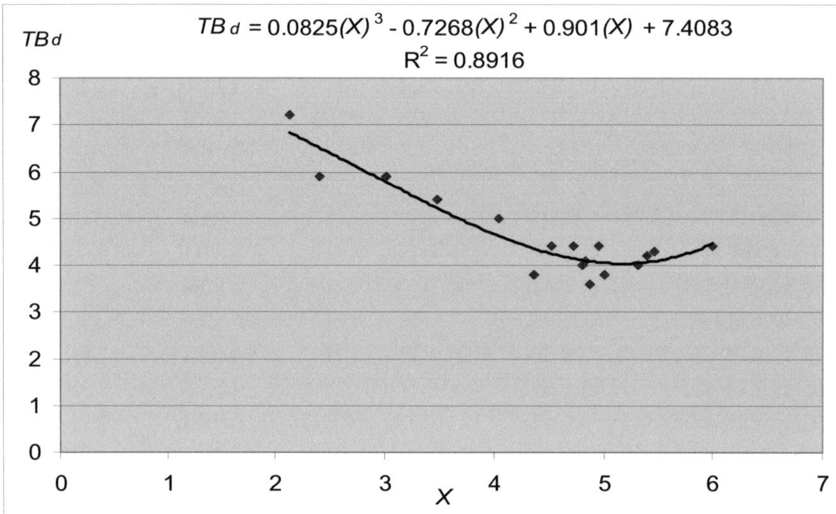

Fig. 3. A curve between values of *Randić* indices (χ) and calculated total biodegradation (TB_d) for **(1-17)**.

By the use of Randic Indices (χ) for **1-17** in the Eq.-4 can achieve to an approximation for total biodegradation (TB_d). All values of TB_d should multiply to 10^{-5} for achieving to calculated total biodegradation in mol/h for the compounds.

A plot of the $\log(K_{ow})$ versus the calculated total biodegradation (TB_d) for Barbiturates **(1-17)** was demonstrated in Fig.-4. The equation of this relationship has three-order structure and introduced by Eq.-5. The R-squared value (R^2) for this graph is equal to 0.9243.

$$TB_d = 0.0286(\log K_{ow})^3 + 0.1884(\log K_{ow})^2 - 1.1251(\log K_{ow}) + 5.314 \quad (5)$$

It seems that two methods were achieved for TB_d calculation of barbiturates **(1-17)**. One of these two models, is calculation of Randic Indices (χ) for these important compounds by the use of Eq.-4.

The second method is the measurement of $\log K_{ow}$ by the use of (χ) in equations 3, then utilize the result in Eq.-5. In respect with the R-squared value (R^2) for these graphs it is obvious that the second model much better for this relationship. Determination of $\log K_{ow}$ and TB_d for the barbiturates as an important class of medicinal compounds have highly importance and the models that were demonstrated here show simple methods for this matter.

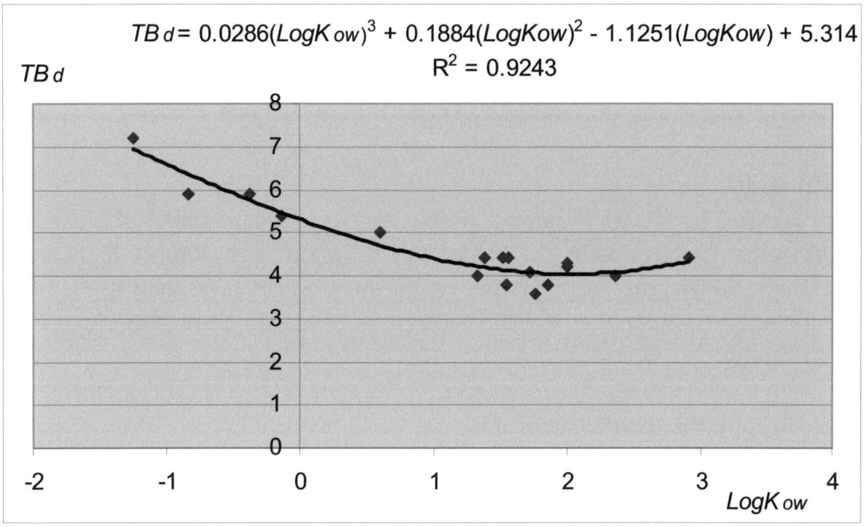

Fig. 4. A plot of the $\log(K_{ow})$ versus the calculated total biodegradation (TB_d) for Barbiturates **(1-17)**.

6. Conclusion

Barbiturates are primarily used for insomnia and preoperative sedation. These drugs contain a "balance" of hydrophilic and lipophilic functionality. General properties of these compounds relatively concern to low *"lipophilicity"* and low plasma protein binding. Graph theory has been found to be an effective tool in *QSAR* and *QSPR*. Topological inices (*TIs*) contain valuable structural information as evidenced by the success of their widespread applications in *QSAR*. One of the useful descriptors for examination of structure-property relationship is *Randić* index. The lipophilicity and toxicity properties of organic compounds can be predicted on the basis of the $logK_{ow}$. The biodegradation QSAR studies demonstrate that microbial biosensors are a viable alternative means of reporting on potential biotransformation. In this study, was considered the relationship of *Randić* indeices, logarithm of calculated Octanol-Water partitioning coefficients and total biodegradation ($logK_{ow}$ and TB_d (mol/h), respectively) with each other for barbiturates. Randic Indices (χ) show a good differences between the values of $logK_{ow}$ and TB_d as two important factors in chemical and biochemical studies in these compounds.

7. Acknowledgment

The authors gratefully acknowledge Dr. Arezou Taherpour for the useful suggestions.

8. References

[1] a) http://en.wikipedia.org/wiki/Insomnia. b) Roth, Thomas (15 August 2007). "Insomnia: Definition, Prevalence, Etilogy, and Consequences" (Full text). *J Clin Sleep Med* (American Academy of Sleep Medicine) 3(5 Suppl) (5 Suppl): S7–S10.

[2] c) Morin, C. M. (2000). "The Nature of Insomnia and the Need to Refine Our Diagnostic Criteria" (Editorial). *Psychosomatic Medicine* **62** (4): 62:483–485. http://www.psychosomaticmedicine.org/cgi/content/full/62/4/483. Retrieved 2010-01-07.

[3] d) Hirshkowitz, M. (2004). "Chapter 10, Neuropsychiatric Aspects of Sleep and Sleep Disorders (pp 315-340)". In Stuart C. Yudofsky and Robert E. Hales, editors (Google Books preview includes entire chapter 10). *Essentials of neuropsychiatry and clinical neurosciences* (4 Ed.). Arlington, Virginia, USA: American Psychiatric Publishing.

[4] e)http://www.who.int/selection_medicines/committees/expert/17/application/Section24_GAD.pdf. Retrieved 2009-01-25.

[5] f) http://www.webmd.com/sleep-disorders/guide/insomnia-symptoms-and-causes.

[6]Insomnia. National Heart, Lung, and Blood Institute. http://www.nhlbi.nih.gov/health/dci/Diseases/inso/inso_all.html. Oct. 7, 2010.

[7] Approach to the patient with a sleep or wakefulness disorder. The Merck Manuals: The Merck Manual for Healthcare Professionals. http://www.merck.com/mmpe/print/sec16/ch215/ch215b.html. Oct. 7, 2010.

[8] Ancoli-Israel S. Sleep and its disorders in aging populations. Sleep Medicine. 2009;10:S7.

[9] Doghramji K. (2010) The evaluation and management of insomnia. Clinics in Chest Medicine. 31:327.

[10] Wortelboer U., Cohrs S., Rodenbeck A., Rüther E. (2002) "Tolerability of hypnosedatives in older patients". *Drugs Aging*, 19 (7): 529–39.

[11] Flamer H. E. (June 1995). "Sleep problems". *Med. J. Aust.*, 162 (11): 603–7.

[12] http://www.dignitas.ch/index.php?option=com_content&view=article&id=22&Itemid=62& lang=de. Retrieved 2011-06-14.

[13] "Barbiturates: How Is It Taken?". *Azdrugs. Org*. 2005–2007. http://azdrugs.org/barbiturates/how-taken. Retrieved 2007-10-31.

[14] Lopez-Munoz F., Ucha-Udabe R., Almao C. (2005) *Neuropsy.Dise.& Treat.*, 1(4), 329-343.

[15] Wallner M., Hanchar J. H., Olsen W. R. (2006) *Pharma. & Therap.*, 112(2), 513-528.

[16] Lanfont O., Talab A., Menager S., Vave C., Miocque M. (1990) *Eur. J. Medic. Chem.*, 25(2), 179-186.

[17] Shimazono N. (1961) *Bitamin*, 24(1), 1-9.

[18] Wasternack C. (1980) *Pharm. & Thera.*, 8(3), 629-651.

[19] For some useful information about Barbiturates see: http://www.duc.auburn.edu/~deruija/GABA_Barbiturates2002.pdf#search='Barbiturates%20structures' and http://www.streetdrugs.org/barbiturates.htm.

[20] Brunton, Laure L.; Lazo, John S.; Parker, Keith L.; Goodman, Louis Sanford; Gilman, Alfred Goodman (2005). *Goodman & Gilman's Pharmacological Basis of Therapeutics*. McGraw-Hill.

[21] a)http://en.wikipedia.org/wiki/GABAA_receptor. b)http://en.wikipedia.org/wiki/AMPA_receptor.

[22] Harrison N.; Mendelson W. B. and de Wit H. (2000). "Barbiturates". Neuropsychopharmacology. http://www.acnp.org/g4/GN401000173/CH169.html. Retrieved 15 July 2008.

[23] Society for Neurochemistry, American; George J. Siegel M.D., Bernard W. Agranoff M.D., Stephen K. Fisher Ph.D., R. Wayne Albers Ph.D., Michael D. Uhler Ph.D. (1999). "Part 2 Chapter 16". *Basic Neurochemistry - Molecular, Cellular and Medical Aspects* (Sixth ed.). Lippincott Williams and Wilkins.

[24] http://www.ncbi.nlm.nih.gov/books/bv.fcgi?rid=bnchm.section.1181.Retrieved July 2008.

[25] Weber, M; Motin, L; Gaul, S; Beker, F; Fink, RH; Adams, DJ (January 2005). "Intravenous anaesthetics inhibit nicotinic acetylcholine receptor-mediated currents and Ca2+ transients in rat intracardiac ganglion neurons."*British Journal of Pharmacology* 144 (1): 98–107.

[26] Chang, Suk K..; Hamilton, Andrew D. (1988). "Molecular recognition of biologically interesting substrates: Synthesis of an artificial receptor for barbiturates employing six hydrogen bonds". *Journal of the American Chemical Society* 110 (4): 1318–1319.

[27] Hansch C., Leo A. and Hoekman D. (1995) *Exploring QSAR: Hydrophobic, Electronic, Steric Constants*, ACS, Washington, DC, USA.

[28] Bundy J. G., Morriss A. W. J., Durham D. G., Campbell C. D. and Paton G. I. (2001) *Chemosphere*, 42, 885-892. (and the literature cited there in).

[29] Hansen P. J. and Jurs P. (1988) *J. Chem. Edu.*, 65, 574-580. (and the literature cited therein).

[30] Hosoya H. (1971) *Bull. Chem. Soc. Jpn.*, 44, 2332-2339.

[31] Randić M (1998) *Acta Chim. Slov.*, 45, 239-252.

[32] Rücker G. and Rücker C. (1999) *J. Chem. Inf. Cmput. Sci.*, 39, 788-802.

[33] Wiener H. (1947) *J. Am. Chem. Soc.*, 17-20.

[34] Du Y. P., Liang Y. Z., Li B. Y. and Xu C. J. (2002) *J. Chem. Inf. Cmput. Sci.*, 42, 1128-1138.

[35] Randić M. (1975) *J. Am. Chem. Soc.*, 97, 6609-6615.

[36] Kier L. B., Hall L.H. (2000) *J. Chem. Inf. Comput.. Sci.*, 40, 729-795.

[37] Estrada E. (2002) *Internet Electron. J. Mol. Des.*, 1, 360-366.

[38] Kier L. B. and Hall L. H. (1976) *Molecular Connectivity in Chemistry and Drug Research*, Academic Press, New York.

[39] For study about the EPI-suit v4.00, See US *Environmental Protection Agency* site: http://www.epa.gov/epahome/docs

[40] Cronin M. T. D. and Dearden J. C. (1995) *Quant. Struct. –Act. Relat.*, 14, 1-7.

[41] Hermens J. L. M. and Verhaar H. J. M. (1995) *QSARs in Environmental Toxicology Chemistry*. ACS Symposium Series 606, 130-140.
[42] Degner P., Nendza M. and Klein W. (1991) *Sci. Total Environ.*, 109, 253-259.